T0150790

CHILDBIRTH IN THE AGE OF PLASTICS

CHILDBIRTH IN THE AGE OF PLASTICS

Michel Odent

Childbirth in the Age of Plastics

First published in Great Britain by Pinter & Martin Ltd 2011
This reprint edition published 2017

Copyright © Michel Odent 2011/2017

ISBN 978-1-78066-388-3

The right of Michel Odent to be identified as the author of this work
has been asserted by him in accordance with the Copyright, Designs
and Patent Act of 1988

British Library Cataloguing-in-Publication Data
A catalogue record for this book is available from the British Library

Printed in the EU by Hussar

Pinter & Martin Ltd
6 Effra Parade
London SW2 1PS

www.pinterandmartin.com

Contents

Introduction to the 2017 reissue

The publication of this reissue is an opportunity to clarify the limits of our topic and to re-evaluate its importance with the passing of time. Let us recall that we have selected one particular perspective to look at spectacular changes in human lifestyles during the second half of the twentieth century. The object of this study is the evolution of medicine, particularly obstetrics, during such a short phase of our history. As a witness of this evolution, I am more and more convinced that the history of plastics is a crucial perspective. We must first keep in mind that the history of plastics started long before the second half of the twentieth century: the world's first fully synthetic plastic was 'bakelite', invented in New York in 1907 by Leo Baekeland, who coined the term 'plastic'. However there were no medical applications until the middle of the century. The first spectacular applications had been military. It is significant that plastics were essential to the building of the atomic bomb at the end of World War II: Manhattan project scientists relied on Teflon's resistance to corrosion.

We must also keep in mind that today, during the twenty-first century, the history of obstetrics is more and more influenced by other factors than advances in plastic technology. It is probable that from now on emerging and fast developing scientific disciplines such as epigenetics, metagenomics bacteriology and epidemiology will be associated with new ways of thinking and will be more influential than purely technical advances. This is why we can present this 2017 edition without any correction or additions.

1

The history of medicine in the light of the history of plastic

It happened on Tuesday November 1, 1949. In the morning of the very first day of my medical studies, I was introduced in the surgical unit of Hôpital Cochin, in Paris. Younger doctors might find it strange that French students my generation were abruptly in touch with the real world before learning from textbooks of anatomy, physiology and pathology. One of the effects of starting a medical career that way is a clear memory of what a huge hospital common bedroom looked like in the middle of the twentieth century. I can remember in particular that during the six months I spent in that surgical unit I never saw a patient whose arm was connected to a bottle.

I became familiar with drips during the first months of 1952, in a medical unit specialising in the treatment of lung tuberculosis. Then two recently discovered effective drugs were routinely associated: streptomycin and PAS (p-aminosalicylic acid). PAS was administered intravenously from a glass bottle via a rubber tube connected to a steel reusable needle. After that, during the winter 1953–1954, I never saw a labouring woman receiving an intravenous treatment during the six months I spent as an *externe* (medical student with limited clinical responsibilities) in the maternity unit of Hôpital Boucicaut. The first obvious reason was that synthetic oxytocin was not available: it was precisely in 1953 that Vincent du Vigneaud established its chemical formula and made its synthesis possible. Another reason was that childbirth was not yet highly medicalised: a maternity unit, even in an avant-garde Paris hospital, was not the right place to detect the first signs of the plastic revolution, although it was the very time when polymer chemists were finding new compounds almost weekly, engineers were constantly improving medical equipment, and ethylene oxide (ETO) sterilization was proven effective and non-harmful to plastics. It is only during the second half of the 1950s, when trained as a surgeon, that I started to realise the importance of plastic in modern medicine.

I participated in a new phase of the plastic revolution when in the French army, during the War of Independence in Algeria, in 1958–1959. The history of emergency surgery always went through spectacular new steps during wars. At that time all the tubes were in plastic. Polyethylene tubes were widely used. I became familiar with the technique of 'venous cutdown', as an emergency procedure making possible massive fast blood transfusions: through a one-centimetre incision at the level of the ankle, the great saphenous vein was exposed surgically and then a polyethylene tube was inserted into the vein under direct vision.

The history of medicine during the past fifty years cannot be dissociated from the history of the use of plastic material. Disposable medical devices developed gradually after 1960. Around 1970 plastic bags were introduced, thus reducing the risk of air embolism. New plastics, less and less traumatic to veins, replaced polyvinyl chloride (PVC). Around 1970, there was the Teflon revolution, followed in the 1980s by the polyurethane revolution. The use of intravenous drips became so widespread in modern hospitals that the procedure of intravenous cannulation became gradually the business of nurses and midwives, while it was originally the business of doctors. Advances in the medical use of plastics have induced a new phase in the relationship between doctors, nurses, and midwives. Today there is a new realm for specialised doctors. It is to introduce plastic tubes in any vessel, in any organ, and in parts of the body that until recently were accessible only through direct surgical routes.

Plastics have transformed most medical disciplines. For example, anaesthesiologists were traditionally experts in the administration of inhaled drugs. After the turning point in the history of medicine they became experts in the use of intravenous and epidural routes: what a mutation! We might establish a catalogue of the numerous medical specialties that were radically transformed by the evolution of plastics.

The development of plastics has not only transformed most medical disciplines; it has also made possible the emergence of new specialties, such as neonatology. In the middle of the twentieth century, paediatricians were occasionally asked to take care of newborn babies. Today neonatologists share the activities of departments of obstetrics and there are intensive care units for newborn babies. In such units most babies are in a plastic incubator, with plastic catheters introduced in big veins and in natural orifices. In general the very concept of intensive care is a consequence of the medical use of plastic material.

The plastic revolution has had spectacular effects in maternity units. It was the prerequisite for the current standardised medicalisation of childbirth. Today it is commonplace to visualise a typical labouring woman as a woman whose arm is connected to an IV plastic bag via a plastic tube, while a catheter has been introduced in her epidural space. People my generation can easily realise that this is an absolutely new situation. When we are in an unprecedented situation, the priority is to phrase appropriate new questions.

2

Unasked questions about the most common medical intervention in childbirth

A labouring woman was inquisitive and even anxious when she received a drip of synthetic oxytocin. The midwife immediately reassured her that oxytocin is not like a drug: it is "natural". Perhaps this is why there are many unasked questions regarding what is undoubtedly the most common medical intervention in childbirth on all five continents. Let us recall that oxytocin is considered the main birth hormone, first because it is necessary to induce and maintain effective uterine contractions for the birth of the baby and for the delivery of the placenta, and also because it may be presented as the main love hormone. Today, all over the world, most women giving birth vaginally get such a drip (called *Syntocinon* or *Pitocin*) including those with an eventual operative delivery by forceps or ventouse. Most women who undergo a caesarean section during labour have had such a drip before the decision to operate, and this drip is usually continued for some hours after the surgery. Even during and after a pre-labour c-section, synthetic oxytocin is included in many hospital protocols to facilitate uterine retraction. Furthermore, the rates of labour inductions are currently high, and induction almost always involves the use of synthetic oxytocin.

Preliminary questions

This new situation raises important questions. We must first wonder why modern women need substitutes for the hormone that is naturally released by the posterior pituitary gland. Is it because their oxytocin system is disturbed? Is the capacity to effectively release oxytocin depleted from generation to generation, as a result of several aspects of modern life, particularly medicalised birth? This is a vital question for the future of civilisation, since the oxytocin system is involved in sociability, capacity to love, and potential for aggression. Is it mostly cultural conditioning in a context of industrialised childbirth? In this latter case the current situation might be reversible. If it is simply a matter of environment at birth, we need to improve our understanding of the birth process. In fact, we must explore the possible contribution of multiple factors.

Other questions address the substances that might cross the placenta and reach the unborn baby. For example, the kind of fluid used to transport synthetic oxytocin. In earlier times, glucose drips were routine during labour. These infusions were not benign because simple sugar molecules rapidly cross the placenta while the mother's insulin – released in response – fails to reach the fetal bloodstream. There is thus a risk of excessive insulin production generated by the baby's pancreas in response to these circulating high blood sugar levels. Extensive research has confirmed the risks of neonatal hypoglycemia.[1-7] These studies led to the replacement of glucose drips during labour by other liquids, such as Ringer's solution. The results of such studies also apply to labouring women without a drip of synthetic oxytocin if they are encouraged to consume sugar or soft drinks. This is not always understood by the natural childbirth groups. Furthermore, if labour progresses spontaneously, adrenaline-type hormone levels are low, voluntary muscles are at rest, and these women do not need added energy.[8]

Can synthetic oxytocin cross the placenta?

When we finally acknowledge that all over the world most women receive synthetic oxytocin while giving birth, we can no longer deny problems arising from the possible transfer of oxytocin via the placenta. One can wonder why it remains an unexplored issue. The main reason, as we have suggested, might be that oxytocin is not considered a "real" medication because chemically the synthetic form is no different from the natural hormone: it is a simple molecule (a nonapeptide). However, the problem is not simple because the amount of oxytocin reaching the maternal bloodstream via an intravenous drip is enormous compared with the amount of natural oxytocin the posterior pituitary gland can release. Furthermore, natural oxytocin is released through pulsations, while synthetic oxytocin is delivered continuously. Another reason for ignoring this issue might be the discovery of enzymes that metabolize oxytocin (oxytocinases) in the placenta. This finding might have led to a hasty, tacit conclusion that synthetic oxytocin does not reach the baby.

Until now, there has been only one serious article published on this subject.[9] A team from Arkansas concluded that oxytocin crosses the placenta in both directions – after measuring concentrations of oxytocin in maternal blood, in the blood of the umbilical vein and umbilical arteries, and also after perfusions of placental cotyledons. More precisely, the permeability is higher in the maternal-to-fetal direction than in the reverse. Eighty percent of the blood reaching the fetus via the umbilical vein goes directly to the inferior vena cava via the ductus venosus, bypassing the liver, and therefore reaching the fetal brain immediately: it is all the more direct since the shunts (foramen ovale and ductus arteriosus) are not yet closed.

Since there is a high probability that a significant amount of synthetic oxytocin can reach the fetal brain, we must investigate the permeability of the so-called blood-brain barrier at this phase of human development. This "barrier" implies a separation of circulating blood from cerebrospinal fluid in the central nervous system. It restricts the diffusion of microscopic particles, including bacteria, and molecules such as oxytocin. However, Australian researchers presented evidence that the developing brain is more permeable to small lipid-insoluble molecules and that specific mechanisms, such as those involved in the transfer of amino acids, develop gradually as the brain grows.[10] In general, there is an accumulation of data suggesting that the blood-brain barrier works in a specific way during fetal life.[11-14] Furthermore, it appears that the permeability of the blood-brain barrier can increase under the influence of oxidative stress,[15-17] that commonly results when a synthetic oxytocin drip is administered during labour.[18] Therefore, we have serious reasons to be concerned if we consider the widely-documented concept of "oxytocin-induced desensitization of oxytocin receptors".[19-22] It is probable that, at a quasi-global level, we routinely interfere with the development of the oxytocin system of human beings at a critical phase for gene-environment interaction. Within the framework of accepted scientific knowledge, we must acknowledge the important role of oxytocin, particularly in sociability, the capacity to love (of others and love of oneself), as well as the potential for aggression (aggression towards oneself and towards others).[23] Interfering in normal reproductive physiology raises critical issues. For example: "Is there a link between the increased incidence of disorders associated with documented alterations of the oxytocin system (such as autism[24, 25] and anorexia nervosa[26,27]) and the widespread use of intravenous drips during labour?" "What will be the impact on the evolution of our civilizations?" We may even wonder if the widespread use of synthetic oxytocin can induce an unprecedented cultural revolution.

Such questions should inspire a new generation of research.

Let us add that twenty-first century technical advances might oblige us to rephrase many questions. For example, it is possible that in the future a drug such as misoprostol (a synthetic prostaglandin analogue given orally) might compete with intravenous synthetic oxytocin.[28]

3

Unsuited birth statistics

Imagine a woman whose labour has been induced. After induction she spent hours attached to a drip of synthetic oxytocin with or without epidural anaesthesia. If there was no use of forceps or ventouse, this birth will be classified as "spontaneous" or "normal" in public health reports and studies published in the medical literature. The drips of oxytocin are obviously considered minor details which are not worth mentioning in statistics. The traditional contents of birth statistics, as established during the preliminary phases of the plastic revolution, must be entirely reconsidered. For that reason many studies are not feasible and, meanwhile, the emergence of the new generation of research we are anticipating is delayed.

The current situation can be illustrated by typical examples, such as the important WHO survey on maternal and perinatal health in nine Asian countries, published in 2010 in an authoritative medical journal.[1] The contrast between caesarean with medical indication and caesarean without medical indication was the only new factor introduced in this survey. Another example is offered by a retrospective study of special educational needs among more than 400,000 Scottish school children.[2] From the report of this study it is impossible to know how often synthetic oxytocin has been used. Another spectacular example is offered by a Chinese study that examined the association between mode of delivery and psychopathologic problems in childhood.[3] The likelihood of such problems was lowest among children born by pre-labour caesareans on maternal request, while it was highest among those born by the vaginal route with forceps or ventouse. Details about the use of synthetic oxytocin would have been useful to interpret such data, since it is plausible that children born after long and difficult births by the vaginal route ending with forceps or ventouse had been exposed to high doses, while, for obvious reasons, those born after pre-labour caesarean have not been exposed to such medications. Interpretations taking into account the use of synthetic oxytocin would not contradict the results of studies comparing cortisol levels in the umbilical cord vein in relation to different modes of delivery.[4, 5]

On the one hand, the classifications of different modes of delivery are not adapted to obstetrical practices any more and, on the other hand, new criteria must urgently be taken into account to evaluate the practices of obstetrics and midwifery.

Towards new classifications

The need to re-establish birth classifications is obvious when exploring the Primal Health Research Database.* Our database specialises in studies that explore correlations between what happens during the primal period (fetal life, the perinatal period and the year following birth) and what happens later on in life in terms of health and personality traits. It is significant that to get some clues about the possible long-term consequences of what happens at birth we cannot rely on the keyword 'oxytocin', which is not productive. We must select more usual keywords such as 'caesarean', 'forceps delivery', 'ventouse' (or 'vacuum'), 'birth complications', 'intrapartum antibiotics', 'breech presentation', 'cephalhematoma', 'fetal distress in labour', 'meconium aspiration', 'nitrous oxide', or 'obstetric analgesia'.

The database offers only two keywords that are strongly related to the use of oxytocin drips. One is 'labour induction', which is occasionally mentioned. This term did not appear in the national birth register in Sweden until 1991, and is

---

* www.primalhealthresearch.com

therefore missing from several valuable Swedish studies. The other keyword is 'uterotonic drugs', which means in practice synthetic oxytocin, and which leads to the only valuable enquiry of the effects of such medications on cognitive development. This has been possible in Denmark, where detailed birth registers were established as early as 1973. More than 4,000 conscripts, born between 1973 and 1975, were tested for cognitive development at the age of 18, and were also given intelligence quotient (IQ) tests at the same time. There were no significant differences, in term of cognitive development, between those born with uterotonic drugs and the others.[6] It is not possible to draw any conclusions from this study for a number of reasons. There was no information on the doses and on the stages of labour: if they were given mostly during the third stage they could not interfere directly with the development of the child. There was a possible selection bias, since nearly 500 men were exempted from the examination for health reasons. Furthermore, both average cognitive functions and the chances of having been exposed to obstetrical drugs that are related to birth order, were factors that were not taken into account.[7] First-born subjects have a higher average IQ than the others, and the use of medical interventions, including oxytocin drips, is much more common for the deliveries of first babies. This is how we can interpret the results of Israeli and Norwegian studies suggesting that conscripts born by forceps or vacuum have a higher average IQ than the others.[8, 9] However, in spite of its limitations, this historical Danish enquiry may be considered the prototype of the studies we are expecting when the contents of birth statistics have been re-established.

Why new criteria to evaluate the practices of obstetrics/midwifery?

For many decades the list of criteria to evaluate obstetrical practices remained unchanged. This list includes the perinatal mortality rates (number of babies who die before the age of a week), the perinatal morbidity rates (in practice the number of babies transferred to a paediatric unit), the maternal morbidity rates (maternal health problems following a birth), the maternal mortality rates and mortality ratio, and occasionally cost-effectiveness. If this list is not enlarged in the near future, we'll reach a time when it will be justified to consider the caesarean as the best way to give birth in most cases. We must keep in mind that the technique of caesarean delivery has been recently simplified, thanks in particular to the work of Michael Stark, from Berlin, who has developed the "Misgav Ladach method". Today it is possible to do a caesarean in twenty minutes with an average blood loss that is roughly the same as for a vaginal birth. When I did my first c-sections in the 1950s, we needed about an hour and we could not start the operation without having at our disposal one or two bottles of blood to compensate for the blood loss. We must add that today, in the age of plastic catheters, most caesareans are not performed under general anaesthesia. The widespread use of regional anaesthesia is another factor that has dramatically improved the safety of the caesarean.

Can we measure the safety of the caesarean?

In general, those who are directly involved in obstetrics regard the modern caesarean as a safe operation. It is significant that many women obstetricians choose to have a caesarean for the birth of their own babies. The point is that it is difficult to express the degree of safety in statistical language. The golden method in medical research in order to compare two possible treatments, or policies, or strategies, is based on randomization: this means that a population is first divided into groups after drawing lots. One group is allocated a treatment, while another group is allocated – at random – another treatment. Then, during a follow-up period, the comparative ratios of benefits to risks for both treatments are evaluated and expressed in statistical language. For obvious reasons one cannot tell a group of pregnant women that they must give birth vaginally, while other women – at random – are told that they must have a caesarean.

However we can learn from randomized trials that were not originally designed to evaluate the frequency of maternal health problems. One is a famous trial involving 121 centres in 26 countries, designed to compare a policy of planned caesarean section with a policy of planned vaginal birth in the case of a breech presentation at term.[10] More than 2,000 women were involved in this trial. It appeared that the rates of serious maternal health problems were roughly the same in both groups. Similar conclusions can be drawn from a study whose objective was to compare planned caesarean versus vaginal delivery in the prevention of HIV transmission in a population of 436 pregnant women.[11]

These findings are reinforced by a large Danish study[12] looking in retrospect at the 15,441 Danish women who gave birth to a first baby in a breech position between 1982 and 1995. Among them 7,503 had a planned caesarean, 5,575 had an emergency caesarean, and 2,363 gave birth vaginally. Contrary to received ideas, the incidence of haemorrhage and anaemia after planned caesarean section (5.7%) did not differ from that after vaginal delivery and was slightly lower than after emergency caesarean (7%). The rate of thromboembolic complications was 0.1% after caesarean. On the other hand the anal sphincter rupture, which is associated with a subsequent risk of anal incontinence, was 1.7% after vaginal birth. It is commonplace to emphasise that all surgical procedures carry an inherent risk of injuries to organs not directly involved in the particular surgery. The risks must be put in perspective. In these series there were just a few cases of bladder injuries (0.1% during planned caesarean and 0.2% percent during emergency caesarean) and a bladder injury can be easily and immediately repaired. Such risks will be still lower with techniques that restrict the use of sharp instruments. In this series it has never been necessary to perform a 'caesarean-hysterectomy' (to remove all or part of the uterus) to stop the bleeding. The risks of post-operative adhesions (and therefore the risks of intestinal obstruction long after) are also very low after the modern caesarean, particularly if no foreign material such as gauze has been introduced in the abdomen. In the near future it might become a routine to instil specific substances in the peritoneum to prevent adhesion formation.

The risks of maternal death are particularly difficult to evaluate. Once more the studies cannot be randomised. In most statistics these risks appear three to four times higher after a caesarean than after a birth by the vaginal route.[13] But the studies are hampered by the fact that the women having caesarean delivery have conditions, pregnancy complications, and delivery complications that are themselves associated with increased maternal mortality. Furthermore, in developed countries, one needs to analyse the outcomes of at least 100,000 births to significantly evaluate the rates of maternal deaths (or 'pregnancy-related deaths'). These difficulties are to a certain extent eliminated since now, in many hospitals in industrialised countries, the routine is to perform programmed c-sections at 39 weeks in the case of a breech presentation at term. Consequently a large number of statistics are now available regarding c-sections that are not related to maternal pathological conditions. In a report of all women in Canada (excluding Quebec and Manitoba) who gave birth between April 1991 through March 2005, the planned caesarean group for breech presentation comprised 46,766 women.[14] No mothers died in this group, while 41 died in the 2,292,420 women in the planned vaginal delivery group (maternal mortality rate 1.8 per 100,000 births: the differences are not statistically significant).

These considerations are based on recent studies conducted in wealthy countries. (The issues are different when considering the case of rural areas of developing countries, particularly in sub-Saharan Africa,[15,16] where the rates of maternal deaths after caesareans can be 100 times higher than in developed countries).

Combining intuitive and scientific knowledge

Whatever the perspective, one can claim today that, in modern well-equipped and well-organised hospitals in developed countries, the safety of the caesarean is comparable to the safety of the vaginal route. Recent spectacular technical advances symbolised by the simplified caesarean are pushing the history of childbirth towards one particular direction.

However there is a widespread intuitive knowledge that the caesarean as the most common way to have a baby is unacceptable. In other words, whatever our background and our sex, most of us feel the need for new criteria, at the very time when it is becoming easier to rationalise what is still eminently subjective. While technical advances are pushing the history towards one direction, scientific advances are pushing the history towards the opposite direction. They indicate the kinds of criteria we should add to the conventional list. They reinforce the intuitive knowledge many of us still have. They provide new reasons to disturb the physiological processes as little as possible.

4

A tool for the future

In the current scientific context, the concept of critical periods of human development is becoming familiar. From all the disciplines that participate in the "scientification of love" we are starting to understand that the capacity to love develops to a great extent through early experiences, and that the perinatal period, in particular, is critical.[1] In other words all those involved in childbirth are prompted to enlarge their horizon; they must learn to think long term and to think in terms of civilisation. This is why I find it necessary to present the primal health research database* as a tool to train ourselves to think long-term and to think in terms of civilisation.

History of a concept

A reminder of the history of the concept of Primal Health is useful in order to realise that until recently we were highly dominated by short-term thinking. In July 1982 I was invited to speak in Oxford at a conference organised by the McCarrison Society. My presentation, entitled 'Childbirth and diseases of civilization', was a preliminary plea for a new kind of research. We were already in a position to suppose that the sudden increased incidence of certain pathological conditions might be related to new powerful ways to interfere with the physiological processes in the perinatal period. At this conference I met Niko Tinbergen, one of the Nobel Prize winners in 1973 as a founder of ethology. He was the pioneer I was looking for since he had explored the risks for autism in relation to how the child was born.

---

* www.primalhealthresearch.com

The correspondence we had afterwards encouraged me to prepare a book about the concept of health and what makes human beings more or less healthy. This is how in 1986, in *Primal Health*, I presented theoretical reasons to suggest that our health and personality traits are to a great extent shaped during the 'primal period', which is the period of formation of human beings during which our basic adapting systems, those involved in what we commonly call health, are reaching their maturity.[2] I included in the primal period fetal life, the period surrounding birth, and the year following birth. The concept of 'primal health research' was introduced to refer to studies exploring correlations between what happens during the primal period and what happens later on in life in terms of health and personality traits.

Today hundreds of studies belonging to the framework of Primal Health Research have been published in a great diversity of scientific and medical journals. The first function of the database is to make them significant by bringing them together. It is only through an overview of the database that we can draw valuable conclusions. For example it is noticeable that when researchers explore a disorder or a personality trait that can be interpreted as an impaired capacity to love (to love others or to love oneself) they constantly detect significant risk factors during the period surrounding birth. Among such disorders we can mention, in particular, juvenile criminality, autism, suicides and other conditions one can interpret as self-destructive behaviours, such as drug addiction and anorexia nervosa. As long as the different ways to give birth are not re-classified, there will be rigid limits to our knowledge of the long-term consequences of how human beings are born.

Gene expression and Primal Health Research

In spite of these limits, we can already learn valuable lessons from the database. Today the concepts of gene expression and critical periods for gene-environment interactions are becoming familiar in the scientific literature. They imply that some genes may become silent without disappearing. We are learning that the time of exposure to an environmental factor responsible for this process of 'epigenetic modulation' may be more important than the nature of the environmental factor. In such a scientific context we have to raise new important questions when studying the genesis of diseases and personality traits (apart from purely genetic diseases, such as Down syndrome, cystic fibrosis, colour blindness, haemophilia, phenylketonuria, Huntington's chorea, sicklecell disease, or Turner syndrome, for example). Until recently the main questions were about the comparative part of genetic and environmental factors and about the identification of genes. Today the most important practical questions are in terms of timing. We need tools to identify the critical periods for epigenetic modulation.

This is how the Primal Health Research Database has been suddenly assigned a new function by bringing preliminary clues about the critical periods for gene-environment interaction in the case of several disorders and personality traits. In a simplistic way, we can already claim that when the development of the capacity to love (to love others and to love oneself) and the potential for aggression (towards others and towards oneself) are concerned, the period surrounding birth appears as critical. On the other hand, when considering the genesis of metabolic types, the critical periods for gene-environment interaction seem more often than not to precede birth. Through overviews of the database, with the objective of understanding better the concept of gene expression, I realised that when two disorders share the same critical period for gene-environment interaction, we should expect other similarities from clinical, pathophysiological and therapeutic perspectives. This is how I looked in particular at the links between autism and anorexia nervosa[3] and also at the links between obesity and Attention Deficit Hyperactivity Disorders.[4]

In fact, at the current preliminary phase of the history

of Primal Health Research, it is often difficult to interpret the hard data provided by epidemiologists. Even when strong correlations are established between events at different phases of human life, many steps are needed before reaching conclusions in terms of the relationship between cause and effects. For example a dozen studies included in the database suggest that in the case of autism the period surrounding birth is critical for gene-environment interaction. Furthermore there are negative findings according to which events preceding birth do not influence significantly the risks (same average birth weights, placental weights and head circumferences at birth, and no influence on the risk of autism of maternal disorders such as pre-eclampsia). The negative findings also include what happens after the birth (mode of infant feeding and nature of vaccinations, in particular). However a prospective study found that exposure to stressors between 21 and 32 weeks of gestation was a risk factor. There is a plausible association between certain emotional states in pregnancy and birth complications. So one can wonder if the causal events are the stressors in pregnancy or the difficult births.

Enlarging our horizons

In order to explore the possible long-term consequences of how we are born, animal models are apparently useless. The reason is simply that among non-human mammals, when the birth process has been disturbed, the effects are too spectacular and too easily detected immediately at an individual level: the mother is not interested in her baby. This is the case of ewes giving birth with an epidural anaesthesia[5] or monkeys giving birth by caesarean.[6] Babies can survive only if human beings take care of them. Millions of women, on the other hand, take care of their newborn babies in spite of powerful interferences.

We can easily understand why it is much more complex in our species. Because human beings speak and create cultural milieus there are situations when our behaviours are less directly under the effects of the hormonal balance and more directly under the effects of the cultural milieu. This is the case of pregnancy and childbirth. When a woman is pregnant, she can express through language that she is expecting a baby and she can anticipate a maternal behaviour. Other mammals cannot do that. They have to wait until the day when they release a cocktail of love hormones to be interested in their babies. We should not conclude that we have nothing to learn from other mammals. They indicate which questions we should raise where human beings are concerned: in these questions we must always introduce the collective dimension via words such as 'civilisation'. This is why today the main questions are about the future of civilisations born by caesarean, or with epidural anaesthesia, or with drips of synthetic oxytocin.

It is therefore necessary to present our database as a tool to train ourselves to reach the collective dimension. It is noticeable that researchers need huge numbers to detect tendencies and statistically significant risk factors. For example, in a study about risk factors for autism, researchers had at their disposal the recorded data from the Swedish nationwide Birth Register regarding all Swedish children born during a period of 20 years (from 1974 until 1993). They also had at their disposal data regarding 408 children (321 boys and 87 girls) diagnosed as autistic after being discharged from a hospital from 1987 through 1994 (diagnosis according to strict criteria). For each case five matched controls were selected. This is how researchers could eventually detect risk factors in the period surrounding birth.[7]

The main lesson of the primal health research perspective is that we should interpret anecdotes with extreme caution. With anecdotes one can support any thesis. Thinking in terms of civilisation also means that those who explore epidemiological studies must first forget their family, their friends, and particular cases as well. We should not be worried about one particular baby who was rescued by caesarean.[8] The cultural milieu can to a great extent compensate for many deprivations. The questions must be raised in terms of civilisation. What will happen in one or two centuries from now if most human babies are born by caesarean?

5

The oxytocin system of
our great granddaughters

It took a long time for the medical community to digest the concept of lifelong consequences of events occurring during the primal period. Concepts introduced in the 1980s were not widely noticed in the mainstream medical literature. This has been the case for 'perinatal programming', a term introduced by Gunter Dorner, a neurophysiologist in East Berlin. This has also been the case for the more practically oriented terms 'primal health', primal period', 'primal adaptive system', and 'primal health research'.

Today we are reaching a new phase in the history of medical culture. The most authoritative medical journals include more and more articles about 'the effects of in utero and early-life conditions on adult health and disease'.[1] The turning point was the introduction of the concept of 'the fetal origins of diseases hypothesis' introduced by the 'Barker group' in Southampton. There are several reasons why this concept can more easily attract the attention of the medical community. First 'disease' appears as a keyword (instead of 'programming', or 'health'). In fact the main reason is probably that the timing is right. It takes time to digest scientific knowledge and to go from knowledge to awareness.

For those interested in the future of humanity:
an inevitable question

Since we have reached this new phase in the history of medicine and health sciences, the time is ripe to prepare the step further. Today, when we mention the need to enlarge our horizon, we focus on the capacity to think of the possible

21

lifelong effects of what happens during the primal period. We also emphasise the importance of the cultural dimension. It is already possible to anticipate that in the near future we will have to take into consideration and even to focus on the possible transmission from generation to generation of the effects of gene expression, that is to say of early experiences. An analogy can help understanding the vital questions all those interested in the future of humanity will become familiar with. It is as if, under the effects of different factors, particularly early environmental factors, some genes receive a label, while others do not. Some labelling processes are now well understood, particularly the process of DNA methylation. According to the label they have been allocated some genes will become silent, while the others will express themselves. This label may be an addition of methyl marks to DNA. This is the process of epigenetic modulation.

To what extent can the labels attached to genes be transmitted from generation to generation? This is the question of the future. In the past we were only thinking of the transmission of the genome. In the future we will need to know about the transmission of the epigenome. The epigenome is eminently dynamic and responsive to environmental signals. In other words we must learn about the inheritance of acquired traits.

Preliminary answers

The inheritance of acquired traits among mammals appears almost obvious when considering the effects of domestication on brain structures and behaviours. Domesticated animals have few opportunities to take the initiative, to struggle for life and to compete. Compared with wild animals, they don't have many opportunities to activate their brain. The side effects can be evaluated in terms of the evolution of the species. In a great variety of mammals such as pigs, sheep, dogs, cats, camels, ferrets and minks, one of the long-term effects of domestication is a significant reduction in brain size.[2] The changes in the brain of a wild creature into that of a highly domesticated strain happen very rapidly in terms of evolution – after only 120 years of domestication, a brain size reduction of about 20% has been observed in mink.[3]

We can already anticipate several avenues for research in order to confirm that the process of gene silencing is inheritable among human beings as well. For example it is possible to compare black people whose ancestors have been slaves and those whose ancestors have not been slaves. The Overkalix study is an illustration of what we can expect from new methods of research. Overkalix is a small isolated agricultural community in northeast Sweden, without access to the sea food chain. This explains why, according to local weather conditions, there have been periods when the food was plentiful and periods of real famine. The study was conducted utilizing historical records, including harvests and food prices. It was observed that the paternal (but not maternal) grandsons of Swedish boys who were exposed during preadolescence to famine in the nineteenth century were less likely to die of cardiovascular disease; if food was plentiful then diabetes mortality in the grandchildren increased, suggesting that this was a transgenerational epigenetic inheritance. A different effect was observed for women: the paternal (but not maternal) granddaughters of women who experienced famine while in the womb (and their eggs were being formed) lived shorter lives on average.[4,5,6] The Overkalix study has already inspired other enquiries regarding the male-line transgenerational transmission of acquired traits in humans.[7]

There are many valuable studies of the effects of the terrible Dutch famine of winter 1944–1945. It was confirmed that the average birthweights of babies whose mothers were themselves in the womb during the famine are comparatively low.[8] In general many advances regarding epigenetic modulation come from Holland. A Dutch team published the results of a twin study aimed at evaluating the amount of variation of DNA methylation in the human population.[9] Through measurements at particular genes (such as locus IGF2) they could demonstrate that DNA methylation is to a great extent heritable (75%–80% for IGF2). In addition, the authors show that age only mildly influences the amount of DNA methylation at this particular locus. To better characterize the influence of environmental factors, DNA methylation at the same locus was measured in 60 individuals who were conceived during this period of starvation and in their siblings born at a different period.[10] The authors show that there is a significant average decrease of 5.6% of methylation at this locus when compared with the siblings. In contrast, 62 individuals who were in late gestation during the same time showed no decrease in DNA methylation. However, these 62 individuals had a birthweight significantly lower than that of a reference population born in 1943 in the same institutions (3,126 g vs 3,422 g). In contrast, the birthweight of the 60 individuals affected by the famine in the periconceptional period was not changed when compared with the same reference population. This observation shows the limitation of birthweight as a proxy with which to investigate early developmental effect of the environment.

A study of the tendency to be thin or fat at birth in fourth to fifth generation South Asian neonates in Surinam also provided highly significant results.[11]

Unanswered questions

If the lifestyle of mammals can have effects transmissible to the following generations, unprecedented questions suddenly become inevitable. The environmental factors to which human beings are now exposed at the time when they give birth and when they are born have never been experienced by previous generations. For the first time in the history of our species, most women do not rely any more on the release of their natural hormones to have babies: either they use pharmacological substitutes, particularly drips of synthetic oxytocin, or they give birth by caesarean. In other words the human oxytocin system has become useless in the critical period surrounding birth. Keeping in mind the analogy of the shrinking brain of domesticated animals, we must wonder if the capacity to give birth could be depleted from generation to generation. It is difficult to explain why the rates of obstetrical interventions are constantly increasing all over the world. The intergenerational predisposition to operative delivery has already been noticed.[12] In the near future we might learn from international comparisons, since the medicalisation of childbirth did not develop at the same time and at the same speed in countries that are pretty similar in terms of standard of living.

One cannot imagine today more vital questions than those related to a possible transgenerational transmission of the capacity to give birth. In practice the questions are about the future of the oxytocin system of human beings. Childbirth is not the only situation that involves the oxytocin system. Oxytocin is the main component of hormonal cocktails released during all episodes of human sexual and reproductive life. We are already wondering why sexual genital dysfunctions are apparently more and more common, and why breastfeeding statistics do not improve in spite of costly intensive public health campaigns. We know today about the role of oxytocin in our capacity to establish eye-to-eye contacts, to interpret facial expression and to be in a situation of trust. In other words we understand the paramount importance of the oxytocin system in the process of socialisation. We present oxytocin as the main hormone of love.

What will be the effects of a weaker and weaker human oxytocin system? What is the future of love hormones? What is the future of humanity?

6

What makes a substance poisonous?

Before the age of plastics

At the time of Paracelsus, about 500 years ago, the answer to such a question could be summarised in three words: "Dosis facit venenum" (the dose makes the poison). Today the answer is more complex. We give a great importance to the concepts of critical periods of human development. We therefore understand that the toxic effects of certain substances are detectable only at precise periods of human life. For example it is through their harmful effects on the development of the male genital tract at an early phase of prenatal life that certain molecules (such as the plastic-related substance bisphenol A) were classified as oestrogen mimickers. The concept of critical period is not the only reason why the question has become more complex during the twenty-first century. We must also take into account that Paracelsus and his contemporaries were exclusively thinking of potentially toxic substances introduced by natural orifices, particularly the oral way. Paracelsus was also considering inhaled substances, since he identified the health effects that metal workers suffered from metal fumes. Today many substances are introduced directly into the body through needles and catheters. This is the case in particular for the widespread use in medicine of intravenous drips as a way to reach directly the bloodstream.

In the age of plastics

Although the issue of what makes a substance poisonous is much more complex than some centuries ago, we must emphasize that the precept expressed by Paracelsus is to a great extent still valid. It is essential to realise that even the most simple and the most necessary molecules can become harmful above a certain dose.

We have already mentioned how a molecule as simple and as necessary as glucose can become dangerous during labour. This is well understood in medical circles, including in the case of "active management of fetal distress".[1] The general rule is to avoid glucose solutions. However, among the natural childbirth movements, it is still commonplace to compare giving birth to running a marathon and to repeat that labouring women need 'energy', without realising that the prerequisite for the labour to establish itself properly is a low level of adrenaline: this implies that the voluntary muscles are rested and that their need for glucose is reduced. The observations by Paterson and colleagues are highly significant.[2] In order to explain their importance, we must recall that when there are ketone bodies in the urine, it simply means that fatty acids have been used as a fuel because there is a shortage of glucose. They found that ketone levels were higher in women who had been starved for twelve hours before an elective caesarean under general anaesthesia than they were for women who had been in labour. This confirms that labouring women spend less energy than those who are only waiting for an operation without being in labour.

Even H_2O, the most vital of all the molecules, can become dangerous if the supplies exceed the needs. It is easy to explain why labouring women are vulnerable to an excessive intake of water. Labour is associated with the release by the posterior pituitary gland of water retention hormones (oxytocin and vasopressin). Mammals do not drink when in labour. This is how we can explain the well-documented risk of life-threatening syndromes of water intoxication when women are routinely encouraged to drink during labour, even when they are not thirsty.[3,4] There is a widespread belief in the natural childbirth movements that the priority is to reduce the risk of dehydration, while the main risk is in fact hyponatraemia (low blood level of sodium) as a component of water intoxication. There are similar risks if too much fluid is brought via an intravenous drip. We must add that the release of water retention hormones during labour can be presented as the solution nature found to keep the bladder empty during labour.

Of course, in the age of plastics, one cannot ignore the toxic effects of phthalates, which are added to plastics such as polyvinyl chloride (PVC) to increase their flexibility, transparency, and longevity. The National Institute of Environmental Health Sciences and the National Toxicology Program began studying phthalates following a discovery that blood stored in PVC plastic bags for transfusions contained significant concentrations of phthalates.[5] The most common phthalate is di-ethylhexyl phthalate, or DEHP. In bags for intravenous drips and tubing, additives like DEHP can make up 40 or 50 percent of the product.

There are several reasons why this issue is critical. The first is that the effects of phthalates on intellectual development have already been demonstrated, in particular by an authoritative South Korean study.[6] The authors found that high urinary concentrations of phthalate metabolites were associated with lower intellectual quotients (IQ) among 667 children at nine elementary schools. The harmful effects of phthalates have also been demonstrated in the extreme situation of premature babies who spend weeks hooked up to multiple types of medical equipment including plastic tubing such as breathing tubes, feed tubes and intravenous tubes that act as a veritable lifeline. The main finding is that such a prolonged continuous exposure to phthalates is associated with excessive inflammatory responses.[7] We must keep in mind that inflammation is known to trigger prematurity diseases such as bronchopulmonary dysplasia and necrotizing enterocolitis. Furthermore, the studies among premature babies in intensive care units have clarified the mechanism of the inflammatory effects of phthalates: they inactivate a white cells factor (PPAR-gamma) that mediates the resolution of inflammation. The important point, according to these studies, is that neonatal white cells (neutrophils) are more sensitive to phthalate-mediated inhibition of PPAR-gamma than adults' white cells.

These studies among school children and premature babies cannot provide definitive answers regarding the common case of women spending some hours with an intravenous drip while giving birth. There is an accumulation of data confirming the transplacental transfer of phthalates among mammals in general[8,9] and humans in particular.[10] Most babies probably receive some amount of phthalates during the critical period surrounding birth. Is this amount negligible or dangerous? What are the possible long-term consequences? It is essential to emphasize that these phthalates pass directly into the fetal bloodstream, with no possibility of degradation in the digestive tract.

It would be feasible to look at traces of phthalates in the urines of women who had just given birth with or without drips of synthetic oxytocin. Interestingly such tests have been used in other human activities, in particular among professional cyclists. This is how the World-Anti-Doping-Agency-accredited laboratory in Cologne demonstrated that Alberto Contador, the winner of the 2010 Tour de France, very probably used autotransfusion before important mountain trials. In practice this means that a certain amount of his own blood was collected and stored before the competition, and then injected back into the cyclist before an important race: there are understandable advantages at increasing the number of red blood cells before a long cycling race, particularly if it is at altitude.

Very sensitive tests today can find a millionth of a gram, or even less, of certain substances in blood or urine. This measurement process is called biomonitoring. In July 2006, an expert committee of the National Academy of Sciences (NAS) published the results of a comprehensive study of biomonitoring. The committee stated that, "In spite of its potential, tremendous challenges surround the use of biomonitoring, and our ability to generate biomonitoring data has exceeded our ability to interpret what the data mean to public health."

Today, even the experts confess that they are in the dark.

The questions related to bisphenol A (BPA), a derivative of the petrochemical benzene, are different, because BPA is not an additive, like phthalates. It is a basic building block of polycarbonate plastics and epoxy resins, such as those used for metal food cans, hard plastic formula bottles, water bottles, dental sealants, safety helmets and glasses, televisions and computers. When plastics are repeatedly washed, exposed to heat and other stresses, the building blocks of the chemical, which are toxic, are liberated. We can claim that we all have BPA in our blood. Furthermore its easy transfer across the human placenta has been demonstrated.[11] It is therefore not surprising that BPA is one of the 232 toxic chemicals found in the umbilical cord blood of babies from racial and ethnic minority groups during a study involving five independent research laboratories in the United States, Canada, and the Netherlands.[12] BPA has been detected in maternal and fetal plasma, placenta, amniotic fluid, and follicular fluid. Several authoritative publications associating BPA exposure with several diseases have led to polycarbonate plastics being banned in the production of baby bottles in some countries and to some manufacturers switching to BPA-free plastics.

It is now well understood that one of the properties of BPA is to mimic oestrogenic hormones. There is an accumulation of data confirming this 'endocrine-disrupting activity', which can have long-term consequences if there is exposure at vulnerable periods of development, particularly during fetal life. This is how one can explain in particular why the male genital tract seems to be in danger. These 'oestrogen-mimickers' undoubtedly interfere with the development of the testis at the very beginning of intrauterine life: more abnormalities of the penis such as hypospadias, more undescended testicles, lower average sperm counts than in previous generations, and more cancers of the testicles. Reports from animal experiments suggest the transgenerational effects of BPA: this will probably become the main reason for concern in the near future.[13,14] These issues are all the more complex since other man-made molecules that did not exist a century ago probably also behave as oestrogen mimickers. This is the case in particular for many widespread families of polychlorinated and polybrominated chemicals such as PCBs (polychlorinated biphenyls) and dioxins.

A turning point in the history of toxicology

We have already emphasized the strong links between the contemporary history of medicine and the history of plastic. We can extend our observation to toxicology, a scientific discipline closely related to medicine. In the near future one of the main functions of toxicology will be to study the effects on early mammalian and human development of man-made molecules, particularly the ubiquitous plastic-related substances.

What we already know about the developmental effects of plastic-related substances may be considered the tip of the iceberg. For example, the present data about phthalates are not sufficient for evaluating the occurrence of reproductive effects in humans: animal experiments suggest that phthalates also have endocrine-disrupting activities.[15] Future research is obviously needed in this field. It should be noted that phthalates occur in mixtures but most preliminary toxicological information is based on single compounds. It is therefore important to improve the knowledge of toxic interactions among the different chemicals of this group.

A necessary avenue for research has been opened up by preliminary data suggesting that phthalates are able to effect meaningful changes in immune function. It is already plausible that exposure to phthalates is a contributor to the increasing prevalence of atopic allergic diseases and asthma.[16] We must emphasize the need for further research regarding in particular the release of phthalates directly into the maternal and fetal bloodstreams during labour through intravenous drips, since, according to animal experiments, comparatively low doses of phthalates have immune effects when non-oral routes of administration are used.

A Chinese study of faulty development of mice testicles induced by maternal exposure to DEHP can help us to realise the real amplitude of the questions related to phthalates release. The authors could demonstrate that it is through an impact on gene expression that DEHP hinders testicles development.[17] We might say that they studied the 'labels' (the epigenetic markers) that become attached to genes during early experiences. Let us recall that according to the label a gene has been allocated, it will become silent or will express itself. The Chinese researchers looked at the best-known 'labelling process', which is DNA methylation. The method they used was sophisticated enough to conclude that it is precisely for a gestational age of nineteen days and also on the third day after birth that DEHP can significantly increase DNA methylation. The results of such animal experiments should be considered seriously since we understand today that the 'epigenome' can to a certain extent be transmitted to the following generation. Should we be worried about the testicles of our great grandsons?

The turning point we are now observing in the history of toxicology is also determined by the urgent need for further studies in the field of plastic-related substances in general, particularly bisphenol A. Until now the focus has been on the oestrogenic effects of this 'endocrine disruptor'. Preliminary animal experiments suggest that in the future the effects of this molecule on the development of all parts of the brain – and not only the parts of the brain involved in sexual differentiation – will become important topics for research.[18] Once more the study of epigenetic markers and of their transgenerational transmissions, in other words the heritability of acquired traits, should become a major preoccupation. From a long-term perspective there is however a difference between BPA and phthalates, since it is easier to legislate about BPA and to ban its use, particularly for formula milk bottles. However it will probably take a long time, whatever the legislation, to eliminate BPA from human milk.[19]

Legislation cannot easily follow the high speed of the history of plastics.

7

If I were the baby

In the age of empirism

There is a typical situation I often had to face during my career. The midwife on duty was calling me because she was pessimistic about the progress of labour, in spite of apparently suitable environmental conditions in terms of privacy, temperature, etc. Should we go on by the vaginal route, starting with a drip of synthetic oxytocin, with the risk of finishing with forceps, ventouse, or hasty emergency c-section? Or, without waiting too long, should we prefer an "in-labour non-emergency c-section"? Since, in such situations, it was impossible to rely on the rationally expressed point of view of the two actors (mother on another planet and baby in the womb), I often took a decision after wondering: "If I were the baby, what would my choice be?"

Starting with such a question I developed gradually a tendency to try first to avoid long and difficult labours by the vaginal route and to be cautious about the use of synthetic oxytocin. I can illustrate this tendency by recalling that the last time I have used the forceps was in February 1965. Of course in the 1960s, 1970s, and 1980s such attitudes could only be based on intuition and clinical observation. Then a visit to a paediatric unit could convince anyone that, apart from prematurity and intra-uterine growth retardation, the most common reasons for transfer during the neonatal period were births after long, difficult and medicated labours by the vaginal route or after a hasty last-minute emergency c-section.

The support of scientific data

Today a great diversity of scientific data can support this originally empiric strategy. When exploring the primal health research database keywords such as 'forceps delivery', 'ventouse', 'cephalhematoma', or 'birth complications' lead to studies that confirm the possible long-term negative consequences of difficult births by the vaginal route. We might mention in particular the authoritative Chinese study assessing emotional and behavioural problems among preschool children aged four to six. Those born after "assisted vaginal deliveries" were at increased risk of psychopathological disorders.[1] On the other hand, the c-section has become an easy, fast, and comparatively safe operation.

When taking account of the many crucial unanswered questions related to the use of drips of synthetic oxytocin, prudence should be the watchword. Lack of full scientific certainty should not be an excuse to maintain the status quo. In other words, as long as knowledge is limited, we should apply a precautionary approach.

It would be of course unrealistic to eliminate overnight from obstetrical practices what is today the most common medical intervention in childbirth. However one can anticipate a first important step by shifting from routine to personalized and selective attitudes in the case of prolonged pregnancy, a very common situation in obstetrics and midwifery.

Should we toll the knell of labour induction?

In some departments of obstetrics, about one quarter of labours are induced. Labour induction usually implies long hours of drips of synthetic oxytocin and can lead to other medical interventions. Such an epidemic of labour induction is related to the dominant routine approach to duration of pregnancy. This aspect of the industrialization of childbirth is rarely, if ever, the subject of discussion.

Modern pregnant women are given a very precise due date. Pregnancies are punctuated by routine medical visits according to an established program. In the age of medicalised prenatal care, the duration of pregnancy is more precisely calculated in weeks rather than months, using the beginning of the last period as the main criterion. Long in advance women are warned that if their babies are not born on a certain date, their labours will be induced. The first effect of such attitudes is that more and more women doubt that they are able to make labour start without the help of doctors.

An induced labour is more difficult than a labour that has started spontaneously. It usually leads to the need for epidural anaesthesia, which more often than not precedes a cascade of intervention, culminating in a vacuum, forceps delivery, or an emergency caesarean. The 'labour induction epidemic' is a factor explaining the rising caesarean rates all over the world.

At the root of this epidemic are statistics. When looking at very large numbers of births, it is clear that outcomes are optimal when the baby is born between 39 and 40 weeks. The outcomes are not as good when focusing on babies born at 41 weeks or after. Such data lead to simplistic conclusions: 'If we routinely induce labour whenever the pregnancy has lasted more than a certain number of weeks (41 in many hospitals), we'll eliminate the risks of fetal distress and even deaths related to post-maturity'.

Are more individualized strategies possible? The answer is yes. I know from personal experience that a selective approach is realistic. The first step is always to try to determine when the baby was conceived, by listening to what the pregnant woman has to say about her private life, the regularity of her menstrual cycles, etc. There are countless anecdotes of women who were adamant that the baby could not have been conceived before a certain date, and that the official calculations should have been corrected. We must accept that a pregnancy is supposed to be nine months from the day of the conception.

After that the principle is simple. If the baby has been in the womb for more than nine months, its condition is assessed on a day-to-day basis. As long as the baby is in good shape, it is possible to wait. From the time daily assessments have started, only the wellbeing of the baby is taken into consideration, whatever the duration of pregnancy. The most common scenario, by far, is that one day labour will start spontaneously and a healthy baby will be born.

Several methods may be combined in order to check that the fetus is not in danger. Firstly, it is easy for a pregnant woman to evaluate the frequency of the movements of the baby in the womb on a day-to-day basis. When there is a dramatic change, this should be considered a warning. It is also easy for medical staff to repeat clinical examinations. The so-called non-stress test (electronic fetal monitoring) is useless.[2,3,4] If the size of the uterus is evaluated every day by the same experienced practitioner (using a tape measure), it is possible to detect a sudden reduction in the amount of amniotic fluid. A daily 'amnioscopy' is a simple, cheap and safe way to check that the liquid is clear. This means that a tube the size of a finger is introduced into the cervix and, thanks to an incorporated light, the colour of the liquid can be evaluated. As long as the liquid is clear and contains some flecks of vernix, the baby is guaranteed to be in good shape. This test, which I have widely used for many years, has never been popular in English-speaking countries, and tends to be forgotten in continental Europe as well.[5]

Today ultrasound scans may be repeated on a quasi-daily basis. As long as there is a sufficient amount of liquid in the uterus, the baby is almost guaranteed to be out of danger. Nowadays most women are offered a great number of ultrasound scans throughout their pregnancy: most of these scans are useless compared with what an experienced practitioner can expect from a clinical examination after listening to the mother-to-be. It seems, on the other hand, that many doctors are paradoxically reluctant to repeat scans when the baby might be overdue. This is precisely the time when scans provide precious data that have huge practical implications. Individualized selective strategies might also lead to re-establish the use of biochemical tests after the so-called due date: a sudden drop in the urinary oestriol levels (and other hormones such as human placental lactogen) is a sign of placental insufficiency. Routine strategies have made these non-invasive tests redundant.

And what if, suddenly, the baby seems to be in danger before labour starts? In my view, in this case, it is wiser to perform a c-section right away. The priority is to avoid a risky last-minute emergency intervention. With such a strategy, labour induction will finally become exceptionally rare and the number of c-sections related to post-maturity will become much lower than if all labours are induced at 41 weeks.[6,7]

One of the drawbacks of the current prevailing strategies is that many women do not spend the last days of their pregnancy in peace. They are obsessed by the date they were given for induction, if their labour has not started spontaneously. They are in an emotional state that probably tends to delay the onset of labour. Some of them try to use non-medical methods of induction. These women do not always realize that any effective method (from acupuncture to nipple stimulation and sexual intercourse) implies that labour may start before the baby has signalled its maturity. There is no natural way of inducing labour. Some methods are undoubtedly unpleasant and even dangerous. This is the case when castor oil or blue cohosh are used.[8]

Tolling the knell of labour induction would be a first step towards a precautionary approach regarding the use of drips of oxytocin. What about the following steps?

8

Reasons for optimism

After thousands of years of beliefs, rituals, and cultural conditioning, understanding the basic needs of labouring women might be deemed utopian.[1] However, since it would be the prerequisite to a significant reduction of the needs for pharmacological assistance during labour, we must first wonder if it is absolutely unrealistic in the scientific context of the twenty-first century. Modern scientific disciplines have already demonstrated their capacity to challenge many aspects of deep-rooted cultural conditioning. This is a reason for optimism. Our optimism will easily be understood if we refer to one of the most important scientific discoveries of the twentieth century. We do not appraise this discovery because it was a sudden accumulation of data provided by a great diversity of scientific disciplines, rather than a breakthrough initiated by the work of one particular research team in one particular scientific discipline.

Let us recall that during a short period of time centred on the 1970s we learnt that a newborn baby needs his or her mother.

Our cultural background

For obvious reasons this is a real discovery since, for thousands of years, in all human societies we know about, mothers and newborn babies have been separated and the initiation of breastfeeding has been delayed. In other words it has been routine for a long time to neutralise the 'maternal protective instinct'. The nature of this universal mammalian instinct is easily understood when one imagines what would happen if one tries to pick up the newborn baby of a mother monkey who has just given birth.

It would take volumes to review all the invasive perinatal beliefs and rituals that have been reported in a great diversity of cultures. As early as 1884 *Labor Among Primitive Peoples* by George Engelmann provided an impressive catalogue of the one thousand and one ways of interfering with the first contact between mother and newborn baby. It described beliefs and rituals occurring in hundreds of ethnic groups on all five continents.[2]

The most universal and intriguing example of cultural interference is simply to promote the belief that colostrum is tainted or harmful to the baby, and that it is even a substance which needs to be expressed and discarded.[3] The negative attitude towards colostrum implies that, immediately after the birth, a baby must be in the arms of another person, rather than with his or her own mother. This is related to a widespread deep-rooted ritual, which is to rush to cut the cord.[4] Several beliefs and rituals can be seen as part of the same interference, all of them reinforcing each other.

Western Europe is not a stranger to these universal rules. In Tudor and Stuart England, colostrum was openly regarded as a harmful substance, to be discarded.[5] The mother was not considered 'clean' after childbirth until the bloody discharge called 'lochia' had stopped flowing. She was not permitted to give the breast until after a religious service of purification and thanksgiving called 'churching'. Meanwhile the baby was given a purgative made from such things as butter, honey and sugar, oil of sweet almonds or sugared wine. Paintings from that time show the newborn infant fed with a spoon while the mother recovered in bed. In Brittany the baby was not put to the breast before baptism, which took place at the age of two or three days. The Bretons of old believed that if the baby swallowed milk before the ceremony, the devil might enter the baby's body along with the milk.

Man's enormous potential for meddling in the newborn baby's relationship with his or her mother is universal.

During the six months I spent as a medical student in the maternity unit of a Paris hospital in 1953, the routine for the midwife was to immediately cut the cord and to give the baby to a help nurse. I never heard at that time of a woman trying to establish a body-to-body contact with her newborn baby. The cultural conditioning was too strong. Everybody was deeply convinced that the newborn baby urgently needed care given by somebody else.

The discovery

This reminder of a universal deep-rooted cultural conditioning is a necessary step to evaluate the importance of the scientific advances of the 1970s. A new generation of human studies was inspired by what we learned about mammals in general. It is significant that Konrad Lorenz, Nikolaas Tinbergen and Karl von Frisch were the joint winners of the Nobel Prize in Physiology and Medicine in 1973. It is thanks to these founders of ethology, and thanks to the work of other ethologists, such as Klopfer,[6] that we became familiar with the concept of critical periods for mother-newborn attachment. In other words we understood that, among mammals in general, there is immediately after birth a crucial short period of time that will never happen again.

The time was ripe to evaluate the effects of immediate body-to-body contact between mother and newborn baby, as an absolutely new intervention among humans. The names of Marshall Klaus and John Kennell, in the USA, are associated with such studies[7], that were also conducted in Sweden.[8,9,10] In parallel other researchers were interested in the behavioural effects of hormones that fluctuate in the perinatal period, particularly oestrogens.[11,12,13] This is also the decade when a sudden interest in the content of human colostrum developed. Until that time 'colostrum' was a fruitful keyword in veterinary medicine, but not in human medicine. In the seventies the focus was on local antibodies (IgA) and anti-infectious substances.[14,15,16] After thousands of years of negative connotations, human colostrum was officially recognised as a precious substance.

In the 1970s we also learned that when there is a free undisturbed unguided interaction between mother and newborn baby during the hour following birth, there is a high probability that the baby will find the breast during the hour following birth: human babies usually express the 'rooting reflex' (searching for the nipple) during the hour following birth, at a time when the mother is still in a special hormonal balance and has therefore the capacity to behave in an instinctive 'mammalian' way. The result of the complementary behaviour between mother and newborn baby is an early initiation of breastfeeding.[17,18] For obvious reasons, nobody knew, before the 1970s, that the human baby has been programmed to find the breast during the hour following birth.

The 1970s was also a period of fast development in immunology and bacteriology. We must give a great importance to the studies about the easy and effective transfer of maternal antibodies (IgG) across the human placenta.[19,20] This implies that the microbes familiar for the mother are also familiar, and therefore friendly, for the germ-free newborn baby. We had reached a new vision of human birth from a bacteriological perspective. We were in a position to understand that the main questions are about the first germs that occupy the territory and become the rulers of the territory. In other words, we were in a position to understand that, from immunological and bacteriological perspectives, ideally a newborn baby needs urgently to be in contact with the only person with whom he (she) is sharing the same IgG.

Immediate implications and long-term lessons

This sudden accumulation of scientific advances had immediate practical implications. One of them was the development of the concept of rooming-in. Until that time it was usually considered convenient to concentrate the newborn babies in the nurseries of the maternity units. Because this concept of rooming-in had the support of scientific data it could also reach countries under communist regimes. As early as 1981, I was invited to speak at a conference about 'rooming-in' in Olomouc, in the ex-Czechoslovakian Republic. It is also in the scientific context of the late 1970s that in Bogota, Columbia, they found that the mother might be the best possible incubator, and they developed what would become 'kangaroo care'.

Although these important discoveries were intellectually acceptable, the cultural reactions were not straightforward. After thousands of years of interferences, it was difficult to accept overnight a free interaction between mother and newborn baby, without any sort of cultural interference. This is how we can explain the translation by the cultural milieu of the scientific message. While we were learning from scientists that the newborn baby needs its mother, the cultural milieu translated: 'the newborn baby needs its parents'. It is noticeable that it is at the very time when these scientific advances started to be influential that the doctrine of the participation of the baby's father at birth suddenly emerged. While Marshall Klaus and John Kennell could publish in 1976 the classic book Maternal-Infant Bonding' in 1982 they had to call the second edition Parent-Infant Bonding.[21]

We have many lessons to learn from this important discovery of the twentieth century. The first one is that scientific perspectives are necessary to challenge thousands of years of cultural conditioning. It is significant that until the middle of the twentieth century, mothers were not expressing the need for body-to-body contact with their newborn baby during the hour following birth: cultural conditioning was stronger than maternal intuition. The second lesson is that when a scientific knowledge has been acquired, its 'digestion' by the cultural milieu can take a long time. In other words it may be difficult to transform knowledge into awareness.

In spite of such difficulties, there are reasons for optimism. If, during the twentieth century, it has been possible to rediscover the basic needs of newborn babies, it does not appear utopian to rediscover during the twenty-first century the basic needs of labouring women. This will be the determinant step towards a precautionary approach regarding the use of synthetic oxytocin.

9

Promising avenues for research

We can already anticipate which avenues for research will make realistic the rediscovery of the basic needs of labouring women during the twenty-first century. After having accumulated a huge amount of data regarding the mechanical and behavioural effects of oxytocin, the goal should now be to apprehend the conditions for its release and to realise at which point it is dependent on environmental factors.

A fruitful physiological concept

To achieve this goal we must rely on well accepted physiological concepts that are not always well digested and that might be studied more in depth. Adrenaline-oxytocin antagonism is a first typical example of such concepts. It simply means that when mammals, including human mammals, release emergency hormones of the adrenaline family, they cannot release oxytocin, the key hormone in childbirth. Everybody knows that mammals release adrenaline in particular when they are scared, when they feel observed, or when they are cold. The conclusions are apparently simple, since humans are mammals: to give birth, a woman needs to feel secure, without feeling observed, in a warm enough place.

Let us take this opportunity to underline that today the crucial step is usually to digest acquired knowledge. In books for the general public a common recommendation given to women who prepare to give birth offers a typical example of difficulties to deeply understand basic concepts. The common advice to be upright and to walk during labour, based on the simplistic idea that gravity can facilitate the descent of the baby, does not take into account that the prerequisite for the labour to establish itself properly is a low level of adrenaline. Let us imagine a woman in early labour who is passive, for example lying down on one side. Such a situation should simply be interpreted as an indication of a low level of adrenaline compatible with an easy progress of labour. To interfere by encouraging this woman to stand up and walk is at least useless. It is probably counter-productive. It can be unpleasant. An analogy with another situation associated with a low level of adrenaline can help understanding how unpleasant it can be: let us imagine that at the very time when we fall asleep we hear a voice saying 'get up and walk'.

The common comment, among the natural childbirth movements, that labouring women need energy like marathon runners and the advice to routinely consume supplements of sugar is also based on difficulties in digesting what we know about oxytocin release in relation to the levels of adrenaline, in other words about the prerequisite for the labour to establish itself properly. When all the voluntary muscles are at rest the needs for glucose are dramatically reduced.

A fruitful complementary concept

While the concept of adrenaline-oxytocin antagonism is perfectly valid among mammals in general, the complementary concept of neocortical inhibition is useful to apprehend the particularities of human birth. Homo sapiens can be presented as a mammal endowed of a gigantic part of the brain called the neocortex. To simplify we can present the neocortex, thanks to which we use sophisticated ways to communicate and create cultural milieus, as the brain of the intellect. During all situations associated with a huge activity of archaic brain structures – such as giving birth and other episodes of human sexual life – neocortical activity has inhibitory effects. Let us visualise a woman in labour with the eyes of a modern physiologist: we focus on the deep primitive brain structures that are working hard to release the necessary hormonal flow, while we visualise the inhibitions that originate in the neocortex.

From a practical perspective the only important point is to understand the solution nature found to overcome the difficulties of human births: it is simply that during the birth process the neocortex must stop working. When our neocortex is at rest, we have more similarities with other mammals. This solution can be easily understood by a core of women who gave birth without interferences. When women give birth by themselves, there is typically a time when they are cutting themselves off from our world. They forget what they learned, what they read, and what their plans were. They behave in a way that in daily life would be considered unacceptable regarding a civilised woman: they dare to scream, to swear, or to be impolite. They speak nonsense. They can find themselves in the most bizarre, unexpected, primitive, often quadrupedal postures. They are as if on another planet. It is obvious that the neocortical control is reduced. This is the prerequisite for an easy birth.

Understanding this concept and the solution nature found to overcome the human handicap in a situation like giving birth suggests that a woman in labour needs to be protected against any sort of neocortical stimulation: this is another simple way to summarise her basic needs. Let us therefore review the main stimulants of the neocortex.

Language is a specifically human stimulant of the cortex. This implies that in situations associated with intense activity of archaic brain structures, such as giving birth, exposure to language should be avoided. In other words the physiological perspective based on the concept of neocortical inhibitions is a way to rediscover the importance of silence. Of course, after thousands of years of culturally controlled childbirth, silence as a basic need cannot be accepted overnight. It is all the more difficult today since many theories that are at the root of 'natural childbirth' movements have reinforced a deep-rooted cultural conditioning and have introduced in the birthing place a guide (a 'coach') who does not hesitate to use language. For that reason the elimination of language has to be gradual. It should be possible to learn first about the particularly harmful effects of a rational language – for example talking about centimetres. An important step would be to avoid asking a question. To try to provide an answer to a question implies an activation of the neocortex. To realise more easily the physiological effects of a question, an analogy with another situation associated with a reduced neocortical activity, such as sexual intercourse, may be useful. Imagine a couple making love. They are in a pre-orgasmic state. Suddenly the woman asks her partner: 'what do you want to eat for dinner?' This neocortical activation can undoubtedly interfere with the physiological processes.

Light is another well-known stimulant of the neocortex. All physiological processes that are associated with a reduced neocortical activity are facilitated by darkness. This is the case of sleep and parturition. Today we can explain why. There is a 'darkness hormone'. Before falling asleep at the end of the day we usually switch off the lights and we close the curtains in order to increase the release by the pineal gland of this hormone called melatonin. One of the effects of melatonin is to reduce neocortical activity. These are important considerations in the age of electricity. We might add that sight is the most intellectual of our senses. It is noticeable that, when women are not influenced by what they read or what they have been taught, they often spontaneously find postures that tend to eliminate all visual stimulation, e.g. on all fours, as if praying. On the day when the concept of neocortical inhibition is well digested, the issues of dim light and visual stimulation during labour will be looked at seriously.

Several situations are associated with an increased neocortical activity. One of them is what happens when we feel observed. It is easy to understand that when we feel observed, we observe ourselves and our neocortex is stimulated: a way to explain one of the basic needs of labouring women. Giving the priority to this basic need – not to feel observed – would have many practical implications. It would suggest, for example, that there is a difference between a midwife staying in front of a woman in labour and watching her, and another midwife sitting in a corner. It would suggest also that it can be harmful to introduce in a birthing place devices that can be perceived by the labouring woman as ways to observe her or to observe her body functions. It can be a camera introduced by the family. It can be an electronic fetal monitor introduced by the doctor. The effects are similar. Rediscovering this basic need will take a long time in the natural childbirth movements, particularly after the recent 'epidemic' of videos of so-called 'natural childbirth': more often than not a labouring woman is surrounded by several persons watching her . . . including a man, plus a camera since there is a video. The birth is presented as 'natural' because it occurs at home, or because the mother is on hands and knees, or because she is in a birthing pool. But the environment is as unnatural as possible.

The perception of a danger is another situation associated with neocortical activity: attention and alertness are needed when a possible danger has been perceived. This is another way to include the need to feel secure among the basic needs of labouring women. This gives an opportunity to underline the links between the concept of adrenalin–oxytocin antagonism and the concept of neocortical inhibition. Adrenaline is usually a stimulant of neocortical activity.

Emotional contagion[1]

There is one particular aspect of emotional contagion that can have crucial practical implications during the birth process. It is essential to realise at which point emotional states associated with a release of adrenaline are contagious.

When a mammal has perceived a possible danger and is therefore releasing hormones of the adrenaline family there is an obvious advantage that subtle warning messages are sent through body language to the other members of the group. It is the same among humans. We all know that we cannot reach a state of complete relaxation when close to a tense person. This also implies that one of the main preoccupations of an authentic midwife should be to maintain her own level of adrenaline as low as possible. It is worth recalling that traditionally a midwife was a woman who spent her life knitting. This is what I realised when I spent six months in the maternity unit of a Paris hospital during the winter of 1953–1954. The value of this traditional aspect of the lifestyle of midwives is easily interpreted today, when taking account of studies of the physiological responses to repetitive tasks.[2] A repetitive task, such as knitting, is a way to lower the levels of adrenaline.

It is probable that in the near future we will give a greater importance to new ways to study the process of emotional contagion. One of the promising approaches is related to the functions of the mirror neuron system. The story started when Italian researchers found that a neuron can fire both when an animal acts and when the animal observes the same action performed by another. Now the concept has been enlarged and appears as a way to demonstrate and objectify the transference of emotions. A large number of experiments using functional magnetic resonance imaging (MRI), electroencephalography (EEG) and magnetoencephalography (MEG) have shown that certain brain regions (in particular the anterior insula, anterior cingulate cortex, and inferior frontal cortex) are active when a person experiences an emotion and when he or she sees another person experiencing an emotion.[3,4,5,6]

It is ironic that today we need such sophisticated investigations to simply conclude that, when a woman is in labour, those who are releasing adrenaline should be sent miles away.

10

Complying with the shyness of oxytocin

At a time when modern physiology can offer such fruitful concepts, we must develop the art of explaining in daily simple language what is essential. Liliana Lammers, a mother of four children and an experienced doula in London, only needs two words to transmit what all pregnant women should understand. She just talks about the 'shy hormone'. It is easy to explain to pregnant women, whatever their background, that the main hormone in childbirth is like a shy person who does not appear among strangers and observers.

Using analogies

Without explicitly mentioning physiological concepts, the use of analogies is a fast and effective way to explain at which point the release of oxytocin is dependent on environmental factors. Other situations than the labours and deliveries of civilised women are related to oxytocin release. Sexual intercourse is an appropriate analogy, since there is no erection and no vaginal lubrification without oxytocin release. As early as 1929, Bronislaw Malinowski, in his study of the sexual life of the Natives of the Trobriand Islands, had noticed that, even in societies where genital sexuality is free, couples isolate themselves to make love, as if they knew that oxytocin is a shy hormone.[1] Breastfeeding can also be used as an analogy, since there is no milk ejection reflex without oxytocin release. An effective advice, in order to overcome difficulties in breastfeeding, is based on the shyness of oxytocin. The milk ejection reflex, particularly during the weeks following a first birth, becomes easier when mother and baby are in a small dark room, with the door closed, and the guarantee that nobody will enter the room.

Since our main topic is the birth of human beings, we can also use the analogy of parturition among non-human mammals. Non-human mammals are apparently following a simple rule: all of them have a strategy not to feel observed when giving birth. They behave as if they knew that oxytocin is a shy hormone.

We can even refer to childbirth in pre-literate and pre-agricultural societies. There has been a phase in the history of humanity when women used to isolate themselves when giving birth, like all mammals. This is confirmed by a great diversity of documents, such as films among the Eipos in New Guinea,[2] written documents about the !Kung San and other pre-agricultural societies,[3] and word-of-mouth reports from Amazonian ethnic groups, such as those transmitted by the Brazilian midwife anthropologist Heloisa Lessa. The concept of a birth attendant is more recent than is commonly believed, although a mother or mother figure was probably around when a woman was giving birth in primitive societies. This was mostly to protect the privacy of the birthing woman against the presence of wandering men or animals. No doubt this is how midwifery began.

How the shyness of oxytocin was gradually forgotten

As soon as childbirth started to be socialised, there was a tendency to forget the shyness of oxytocin. An alteration of the role of the midwife has been an important step in the socialisation of childbirth. While originally the midwife was the mother of the labouring woman – or an aunt or a grandmother – protecting the birthing place, she became more and more the person controlling the event, the expert guiding the mother-to-be, and also the agent of the cultural milieu transmitting specific beliefs and rituals. Traditional midwives use procedures transmitted from generation to generation. Some of them may be invasive, such as the dilation of the cervix with a finger, or the compression of the abdomen to facilitate the descent of the baby. In many societies midwives try to influence the speed of labour in a traditional way with the use of herbs.

An important step in the socialisation of childbirth occurred on the day when women gave birth in the place where they were spending their daily life. Home birth is comparatively recent in the history of mankind.

The masculinisation of the birth environment

Until the middle of the twentieth century, it was apparently still understood that oxytocin is less shy in a female than in a male environment. Despite thousands of years of culturally-controlled childbirth and in spite of the indirect influence of male medical men, childbirth had remained 'women's business'.[4] Around 1950, in the case of home birth, the doctor – usually a general practitioner – was called at the last minute to use forceps or to witness a disaster. The husband was either in the pub, or the café, or he was given a task such as boiling water for hours. At that time, even for a hospital birth, the environment was still eminently female. The 'knitting midwife' was the central person in the maternity unit.[5] There was a very small number of specialised doctors who were almost invisible, appearing suddenly if the midwife called them for a forceps delivery, and disappearing as quickly as possible after the birth. In the maternity unit where I was an *externe* in 1953–1954 the doctor in charge spent only minutes in his office every morning, listening to a fast report of what had happened during the previous twenty-four hours and, occasionally, talking with the medical students. As a male medical student, I did not dare enter a room where there was a woman in labour. I could only appear during the second stage, because I was supposed to learn the use of forceps. Of course, at that time, nobody could even imagine that the baby's father might be introduced in the maternity unit.

It was just after the middle of the twentieth century when the atmosphere started to be 'masculinised'. The number of doctors specialised in obstetrics increased at lightning speed, and almost all were men. Later on, during the second half of the century, other specialised doctors were introduced into the birth environment, such as neonatologists and anaesthesiologists. Around 1970 an occasional woman made a new demand (as a way to adapt to the 'industrialisation of childbirth') for the participation of the baby's father at birth. It became almost overnight a doctrine supported by theories: the participation of the baby's father at birth became within some years an undisputed 'rule'. At the same time, sophisticated electronic machines invaded the delivery room: high technology is a male symbol. There was such indifference to the gradual masculinisation of the birth environment that there were no serious discussions when midwifery schools started to accept male pupils. Furthermore most schools adopted such selection criteria that in some countries a young man with a good scientific background could more easily be selected than a mother of three. There are countless stories of women who gave birth (or, rather, were delivered) under the control of an electronic machine, in the presence of the baby's father, a male midwife, and a male doctor. The almost total masculinisation of birth had been achieved. All the aspects of the shyness of oxytocin had become completely ignored.

A strengthened cultural conditioning

Until recently, beliefs and rituals transmitted from generation to generation had been the main factors at the roots of cultural conditioning. Unprecedented and sophisticated new factors appeared some decades ago. The transmission of theories considered scientific is one of them. It became fashionable to teach women how to give birth, and particularly how to breathe during labour and delivery. This is how the disciples of Pavlov created the Russian 'psychoprophylactic method' which aimed to eliminate the pain of childbirth. The French obstetrician Lamaze introduced this method into Western countries. In the USA it became known as the 'Lamaze Method'. It was based on the concept of conditioned reflexes. Its main theoretical basis was that the pain of labour is not physiological, but reflex-conditioned. The promoters of this method had understood that conditioned reflexes are related to the activity of the neocortex (the seat of all inhibitions), but they had not understood the solution Nature had found to overcome difficulties in childbirth. They had not understood that a reduction in the activity of the neocortex is the most important aspect of birth physiology among humans. They had not understood that a woman in labour must be protected from any sort of neocortical stimulation and that she must forget what she learned. Instead they thought that pregnant women needed to be reconditioned through education and that labouring women needed to be guided via the use of language.

Directly or indirectly, the influence of this method based on the work of theorists has been – and still is – enormous all over the world. Instead of identifying the basic needs of women in labour in order to facilitate labour and delivery and to reduce the needs for drugs and intervention, the focus in recent decades has been on the elimination of pain and fear via psychological 'methods'. The ambition of some obstetricians was to attach their name to such 'methods', in the same way that practitioners of previous generations were proud to give their name to different kinds of forceps. New actors entered the birth territory: helpers, guides, 'coaches', physiotherapists, psychologists and in French 'monitrices d'accouchement sans douleur' (which means 'monitors of pain-free confinement'). The conditioning of new generations of mothers was that women were not able to give birth without the guidance of an expert. The word 'privacy' was ignored. The socialisation of childbirth had entered a new phase in its long history. We had reached another step farther from the concept of the 'shy hormone'.

Today, in the age of spectacular technical advances directly or indirectly related to the history of plastic, visual messages have suddenly become the main factors influencing cultural conditioning. The power of videos and photos of so-called natural childbirth is enormous. It tends to reinforce the effects of thousands of years of culturally controlled childbirth. Can the physiological language and concepts such as 'oxytocin as a shy hormone' reverse this unprecedented extreme situation?

The highest possible peak of the shy hormone

These general considerations about the 'shy hormone' must be completed by questions about what is probably the highest possible peak of oxytocin a woman can release during her whole life. The team headed by Kerstin Uvnäs-Moberg have demonstrated that just after giving birth a mother has the capacity to reach a level of oxytocin that is still higher than for the delivery itself.[6] This peak is vital since it is necessary for a safe delivery of the placenta with minimum blood loss, and also because oxytocin is the main love hormone.

Knowing that oxytocin release is highly dependent on environmental factors, we must wonder what kind of environment can influence this special hormonal peak just after the birth of the baby. The first condition is that the mother is not cold. Regina Lederman found that the level of adrenaline can return to normal as early as three minutes after birth.[7] She has therefore demonstrated how crucial this short period of time is, and confirmed what can be learned from clinical observation. When asked what to prepare for a home birth, I only talk about electric radiators and extension cords, so that warm blankets or towels are constantly available. If a woman is shivering just after the birth of the baby, it simply means that she is not warm enough.

The second condition is that the mother is not distracted when discovering her baby. The mother needs to feel the contact with the baby's skin, to look at the baby's eyes, and to smell the odour of her baby. Any distraction can bring her back to our planet and inhibit the oxytocin release. This is how one can explain the skyrocketing rates of maternal deaths related to postpartum haemorrhages in ethnic groups where the rituals are particularly invasive. It would take volumes to mention all the possible ways to distract the mothers just after the birth. A typical widespread interference is to rush to cut the cord. It is an obvious distraction. It will take time to digest these simple rules that have been ignored for ages. Meanwhile, it is recommended to rely on a substitute for the natural oxytocin to facilitate the delivery of the placenta. It is currently the best way to save lives. This is particularly important in developing countries where a specific drug (misoprostol) is cheap, can be stored at room temperature, and does not need to be injected. It takes ten minutes to learn how to use misoprostol. It will take decades to reverse thousands of years of deep-rooted cultural conditioning and to understand the concept of the love hormone.

If...

If we assimilate valuable lessons from the most promising avenues for research expressed with the language of physiologists...

If we realize the importance of the concept of the 'shy hormone'...

We can reach a radically new understanding of childbirth. The first stage of labour can be presented as the phase preceding the fetus ejection reflex. The fetus ejection reflex is a short series of irresistible powerful contractions preceding the birth of the baby. During a fetus ejection reflex there is no room for voluntary movements. This term has been used originally by Niles Newton in her studies of the birth of mice.[8] I found it relevant to use it for human beings, who have more similarities with non-human mammals when their neocortex is at rest.[9]

The fetus ejection reflex is not easily understood after

thousands of years of cultural interferences, because the conditions that make it possible are uncommon in our societies. One of the usual ways to interrupt the process leading to a fetus ejection reflex is to use language when there is an obvious elimination of neocortical control, for example when the labouring woman suddenly says: 'kill me', 'shoot me', 'let me die', 'do anything', 'my bowels are going out . . . do a caesarean', etc.

Because basic simple rules are not well digested, the fetus ejection reflex is more often than not transformed into a second stage of labour, with a need for voluntary movements.

A real fetus ejection reflex is compatible with an ecstatic/orgasmic state, often described afterwards as a transcendent emotional state. The climax can be reached just after the birth, at the time of the first eye-to-eye contact between mother and newborn baby. It is noticeable that all cultural milieus have made this route to transcendence impossible.[10]

When there is an authentic fetus ejection reflex, the midwife can forget her usual worries about, for example, shoulder dystocia, difficulties for the delivery of the head in the case of a breech presentation, difficult process of rotation, dangerous perineal laceration, etc.

Understanding the art of midwifery as the art of creating the conditions for a fetus ejection reflex would pave the way for a real paradigm shift. For thousands of years cultural milieus have more or less controlled the physiological processes related to childbirth. They have done that in particular by transmitting the deep-rooted belief that a woman has not the ability to give birth without the assistance of a helper: to help is a subtle way to control. This conditioning is still basically the same in medical and midwifery circles, and in natural childbirth movements as well. The main lesson of modern physiology is that the process of parturition is an involuntary process related to the activity of archaic brain structures. One cannot help an involuntary process, but certain situations can disturb it. This leads to realise that labouring women do not need direct active help. They need mostly protection against any factor that might increase the levels of adrenaline or stimulate the neocortex. Are we at the dawn of such a necessary new paradigm?

11

Learning from home births

Introducing a more precautionary approach with regard to pharmacological assistance in childbirth leads also to look at what we can learn from out-of-hospital births, compared with births in conventional departments of obstetrics. It seems easy to analyse the reasons why most labouring women need pharmacological assistance (particularly drips of synthetic oxytocin and epidural analgesia) in hospital settings. It may appear a priori more difficult to acknowledge and to interpret the common difficulties of home births and therefore simply conclude that modern women in general have difficult births.

Authoritative studies

The difficulties of home births have been evaluated by an authoritative meta-analysis (combining data provided by several studies using similar protocols) published in *The American Journal of Obstetrics and Gynecology*.[1] All the studies in this article had compared the outcomes of planned home births with planned hospital births. This being the best method since randomised controlled trials are not feasible. Let us recall that studies comparing outcomes of actual home with actual hospital births underestimate the risks associated with planned home births, because they do not take into account the transfers to hospital during labour. The studies included in the meta-analysis had been conducted in developed western countries (USA, UK, Canada, Australia, Switzerland, Netherlands, and Sweden) and published in the English language in peer-reviewed medical journals.

Among the results provided by this meta-analysis we

must keep in mind one significant statistics. It is noticeable that, in the planned home birth group, up to 37% of women giving birth to their first baby require transfer to a hospital during labour. It is also noticeable that the neonatal death rates (deaths between birth and the age of 28 days) appear twice as high after planned home births than after planned hospital births, and almost tripled among newborn babies without abnormalities.

The data provided by a recent study covering the whole region of Utrecht, Holland, are particularly thought-provoking because they might lead to a reconsideration of the very special Dutch system. This system is different from all other obstetric care systems because it is based on a well-defined distribution between primary and secondary care. In practice women with a low risk of pathology are in the hands of midwives, while the others are in the hands of obstetricians. One of the effects of this classification is a rate of home birth still above 25%. According to this study, the risks of perinatal death are significantly increased when the pregnancy was classified as low risk.[2]

The results of these studies are not surprising if one takes into account the widespread lack of understanding of the basic needs of labouring women conveyed in particular by certain natural childbirth movements. As we have already noticed, this lack of understanding has been recently reinforced by the power of visual messages, particularly the current epidemic of videos showing a woman giving birth surrounded by two or three persons watching her (including a man, plus a camera). We have previously commented on these births that are called 'natural' because they occur at home, or because the woman is on hands and knees, or because she is in a birthing pool. But the environment is as unnatural as possible.

These visual messages strengthen the deep-rooted cultural conditioning that a woman only has the power to give birth when surrounded by people bringing their energy ('support') or their expertise ('coach'). This is exactly the opposite of the correct message: 'to feel secure without feeling observed' is a basic need during labour. The difficulties of home births in our societies underline how urgent it is to rediscover the basic needs of labouring women. Meanwhile one can anticipate that in the near future home births will become even more difficult. Until now the time periods covered by published studies did not go beyond 2006, apart from the Dutch study, which covered the years 2007 and 2008. We will constantly need updated studies with quite similar protocols.

An overview of obstacles to overcome

After being involved in childbirth for more than half a century in hospitals, at home, and in different countries, and after taking into account what we can learn from the physiological perspective, I feel authorised to indicate the main obstacles that should be overcome to make home births much easier and therefore safer. Referring to these obstacles is a different and indirect way of repeating what we already know about the basic needs of labouring women.

An important first step will be to challenge the deep-rooted cultural belief that a woman is unable to give birth by herself. One of the practical effects of this belief is that if by chance a woman is giving birth so easily that she cannot reach a hospital or cannot have the assistance at home of a birth attendant, the birth is bound to occur in an atmosphere of panic rather than euphoria or joy. It should be easy to explain in advance that such easy unmedicated births are usually safe, and convince anyone that there is nothing urgent to do, apart from making sure that mother and baby are not cold. Getting rid of this belief would make unplanned home births (or births in an unexpected place at an unexpected time) as safe as possible.

One of the main obstacles for easy births – particularly easy home births – is the common overuse of language. I have countless anecdotes of useless questions, comments, and advices by well-intentioned birth attendants.

Another obstacle is a deep-rooted tendency to introduce without any caution several people around the labouring woman. This tendency is as old as the socialisation of childbirth. In many societies one of the women around plays the role of the midwife, often accompanied by relatives or neighbours. Traditionally the midwife is an autonomous, very independent person. There are proverbs, in places as diverse as Persia or South America, claiming that the presence of two midwives makes the birth difficult. In Persia, they used to say: "When there are two midwives, the baby's head is crooked".[3] Such widespread observations are easily interpreted when keeping in mind that the midwife is originally the mother, or the substitute for the mother: it is difficult to rely on two mother figures at the same time.

New ways to multiply the number of birth attendants have recently been introduced. Some of these new ways have even been officialised. For example, when a British woman wants to stay at home for the birth of her baby and calls the community midwives of the National Health Service, the rule is to send a pair of midwives. Those who have established such rules could not imagine that it might be a way to make the births more difficult and therefore less safe. Not only is the presence of two midwives more and more common, but also today another birth attendant, a doula, may be introduced in the birthing place. The doula phenomenon is such a sudden international phenomenon that it must be analysed and interpreted in the context of the twenty-first century.

The doula phenomenon

The doula phenomenon can be presented in a positive or in a negative way. This is why it is necessary to refer to the emergence of the phenomenon. The story started in the 1970s in two busy hospitals in Guatemala, where fifty to sixty babies were born every day and where the routines

MICHEL ODENT

had been established by doctors and nurses from the United States. There were no midwives. It is in such a context that John Kennell and Marshall Klaus evaluated the effects of the presence of a lay female companion during labour. The female companion was simply a mother who lived nearby who had had the experience of giving birth. It appeared that the presence of such a mother figure in the context of a busy Latin American hospital was a way to make the births easier and therefore to improve the statistics. The results of these studies were published in mainstream medical journals.[4,5] In these published articles the female companion was called a 'doula': the authors had been told that in ancient Greece the doula was a servant taking care of the labouring woman. These studies were reproduced in Houston, Texas, in a neighbourhood where the population is predominantly Hispanic and incomes are low. There, the birth care-givers were directed by English-speaking residents in a twelve-bed ward. The doulas spoke both Spanish and English. As in Guatemala, the presence of a doula brought positive effects.[6]

As long as the studies were conducted in low-income Hispanic populations, the statistical results clearly confirmed the positive effects of the presence of a doula. The findings were different in the context of middle-class American populations such as the Kaiser Permanente Care program of Western California, where the presence of a doula had no impact on the rates of caesarean deliveries and other operative deliveries.[7] Such differences need to be interpreted. One of the many differences is that at Kaiser Permanente the baby's father was almost always present. Unfortunately the authors of the report did not provide any information about the way the doulas had been chosen. They found it more important to underline that all of them attended approved training programmes and had served as doulas for at least two births under the supervision of a more experienced doula (supervising a doula is a powerful interference!). One can wonder if the training might not be counter-productive. Once I had dinner with three of the doulas who were

64

involved in the Houston study. They spoke a lot about the birth of their own children as positive experiences. They never mentioned any 'training'. The term "training' suggests that what the doula does is more important than who she is. These discrepancies in the results remained unnoticed. This is how the word doula has been introduced into the American vocabulary.

Personally I thought originally that there was a reason for doulas in the USA, but not in countries where there were many midwives, particularly in Western Europe. However, in 1998, I was asked to do information sessions for doulas in London. Then I understood the reasons for doulas even in a country like the UK. After meeting several prenatal health care professionals, after experiencing the effects of the midwives' shifts during labour, and after meeting several other health professionals for postnatal care, many women started to realise that there was indeed something wrong in the system. They were feeling the need to rely on the same mother figure before, during, and after the birth. At the same time some women who had already gone through the experience of giving birth felt the need to protect younger ones. Many of these women were typical mother figures.

When I associated with Liliana Lammers, an experienced doula, for such sessions, we had to clarify the vocabulary. Having studied ancient Greek, I was not comfortable with the word 'doula', which in fact means 'slave'. We also had to take into account the importance of the Greek community in London. Greek friends advised us to use the word 'paramana', which means literally 'with the mother'. This is how we adopted the term 'paramanadoula course', combining a term accepted by the Greek community and a term internationally used. We refer to 'information sessions', avoiding the term 'training'. Of course a doula needs to be informed. With a well-informed doula, the young mother feels more secure. An ideal doula must be aware of everything related to pregnancy, childbirth and breastfeeding, even if her knowledge is superficial.

The doula phenomenon must be interpreted in the context of a period of transition. It might be a step towards a 'demasculinisation' of the birth environment. There are already stories of women who prefer going to the maternity unit with a female friend who has had babies than with their husband/partner who is out of context. When the doula is understood as the mother figure a young woman can rely on before, during and after the birth, the doula phenomenon can be presented in a positive way as an aspect of the rediscovery of authentic midwifery. When, on the other hand, the doula is yet another person introduced into the birthing place in addition to the midwife, the doctor and the father, her presence is counterproductive. If the focus is on the training of the doula rather than on her way of being and her personality, the doula phenomenon will be a missed opportunity.

The participation of the baby's father at birth

The doctrine of the participation of the father is another modern way to multiply the number of birth attendants. It is probably the most difficult obstacle to overcome in order to make home births easier, although originally the doctrine was not related to home births. As with the doula phenomenon, it was originally related to the 'industrialisation' of childbirth. It started with an occasional unexpected demand by some labouring women who wanted to keep the baby's father with them. It was an understandable attempt to adapt to the concentration of births in huge hospitals, since the baby's father – usually the driver of the car – was a familiar person. It was difficult to anticipate at what speed this occasional demand would be transformed into a doctrine. Theoreticians only took into account the anecdotal enthusiastic reports of positive experiences without realising the complexity of the issue. We heard that the participation of a familiar person should make the births easier and should lead to a decreased need in medical intervention. We also heard that the participation of the father should reinforce the links between the couples to the extend that divorces would become less common. Since it was the beginning of 'The Scientification of Love', with the popularisation of the word 'bonding', we heard more and more about the 'bonding' between the father and the newborn baby, as if it could be symmetrical to the bonding between mother and baby.

Today we can at least claim that if the physiological processes had been better understood when the dogma was being established, theoreticians would have been more cautious. If they had been aware of the adrenaline-oxytocin antagonism, if they had anticipated that, in such situations, when a man loves his wife he can reach high levels of stress hormones, and if they had known at what point the release of stress hormones is contagious, the participation of the baby's father would have remained occasional.[8]

Let us dare to smash the limits of political correctness and wonder if the usual participation of the father is one of the main factors explaining the difficulties of modern births, particularly home births.

I am convinced that the best possible environment for an easy birth is when there is nobody around but an experienced and silent midwife or doula, perceived by the birthing woman as a mother figure. I learned this at the time of the 'knitting midwife' – in the early 1950s. I am relearning this today when, occasionally, I attend a home birth, and keep the baby's father busy in the kitchen or elsewhere around the house, thus leaving the labouring woman with only one person around – an experienced, motherly and silent doula. However, in the present age of evidence-based obstetrical and midwifery practices we cannot rely on clinical observation to provide an answer. At the same time, the 'golden method' cannot evaluate the effects of different degrees of masculinisation of the environment upon the birth process and upon the first contact between mothers and newborn babies. That is, randomised controlled trials

(RCTs) are not feasible. This is why international comparison is one of the best approaches.

International comparisons are valuable because the participation of the father, although an international phenomenon, did not occur simultaneously and at the same speed in different countries. Number one among countries where masculinisation started early and developed at a high speed was the USA. In the USA, the doctrine of the husband/partner participating in the birth was already well established in the early 1970s. At the other end of the spectrum, the masculinisation process has been delayed in a certain number of countries. For instance, obstetrics in Ireland is usually associated with the concept of 'active management of labour', using strict pre-established criteria to control the speed of labour. Yet, the history of obstetrics in Ireland has another characteristic: the routine presence of the father in Irish births was delayed until the late 1980s. The unique characteristic of the socialised Dutch system of midwifery and obstetrics is that the midwife is officially considered the *primary care giver*. The obstetrician plays the role of the expert adviser on demand. Until recently Holland has not been highly influenced by the theories of most Western natural childbirth movements. There, the traditional behaviour of the husband going to the pub or being busy in the house persisted longer than in other countries. The concept of the *couple* giving birth appeared much later than in other Western European nations. Outside Western Europe, Russia is a country where the masculinisation process has been delayed. Until recently fathers were not permitted to enter the maternity units. In 1992, I saw a mother showing her baby to her husband through the window of a maternity unit in Moscow, while he had to stay outside, in the street. Now, suddenly, all aspects of the Western lifestyle are becoming widespread in Russia, affecting the birth environment, and the participation of the father is more and more common.

Ireland, Holland, and Russia share another common

point. The spectacular ascendance of caesarean sections has been delayed as well. The incidence today tends to be similar to elsewhere. Of course, in order to interpret this correlation, we must take into account that in some particular cultural milieus the inhibitory effect of a male environment might be stronger than in others. This might be the case, for example, in Southern Italy, a region influenced by Arabic cultures, where the rates of caesareans are skyrocketing.

Beyond the birth

When trying to assess the safety of home birth in relation to the participation of the father, we should go beyond the birth itself. We must also consider the health of the father in the days following the birth. At a time when I was attending home births by myself – a time when the dogma of the father participating in the birth was unchallenged – I became aware of this issue. When visiting the family some days after a birth, I often found the mother happy and active with her baby. At the end of my visit I used to politely ask news about the rest of the family. This is how I realised that health problems in the father are common during the days following modern home births. There was almost always a rather precise diagnosis, such as lumbago, kidney stones, generalised eczema, abdominal pain, or toothache, for example. The timing of these diseases was always presented as 'bad luck'. Without asking questions I would have missed these health problems apparently unrelated to the birth. My list of such anecdotes became longer and longer when I started discreetly inquiring into these issues. The interpretation I suggest is that all these health problems might be considered as different facets of 'male postpartum depression'.

Depression in men is largely unacknowledged and unrecognised because it is usually 'masked' by a great diversity of misleading symptoms. According to Terrence Real, who coined the term 'covert depression', we tend not to recognise depression in men because the disorder itself is seen as unmanly.[9] Depression carries, to many, a double stain – the stigma of mental illness and also the stigma of 'feminine' emotionality. Depression is hidden from the men who suffer from it and also from those who surround them.

My interest in the health of the baby's father in the perinatal period also led me to consider the strange behaviour of some of them in the days following a modern type of unmedicated birth. One disappeared the day after the birth and went back to his native country. Another had an urgent unexpected need to spend his day playing golf. Another one could not stop playing computer games. We can introduce in the same framework the case of a man who had his first attack of schizophrenia at the age of thirty-five two days after the birth of his baby. The behaviour of all these men had been 'normal' – according to modern books – on the day of the birth. Obviously all these men felt the need to escape from daily reality, one way or another. Modern physiology can explain that, in adverse circumstances, there are two ways to protect our health: 'fight or flight'. These men had an urgent need to protect their health by escaping.

A man I had known personally paid an extreme price for the strong emotional reactions he experienced during a 'wonderful' out-of-hospital birth – a birth in the ocean. This man died from a heart attack when the baby was just a few days old.

Why focus on home birth?

In Western developed countries (apart from the Netherlands) at least 97% of babies are born in hospitals. However we have good reasons to give a great importance to out-of-hospital births. If out-of-hospital births were made easier, we might expect that, through a process of 'osmosis', hospital births would become easier as well, and furthermore there would be more home births. In other words we should expect a significant step towards a precautionary approach with regards to pharmacological assistance during labour and particularly the use of synthetic oxytocin.

Reconsidering old rituals in order to facilitate certain phases of labour, such as the phase between the birth of the baby and the delivery of the placenta, would have impacts in developing countries as well. Cutting the cord before the delivery of the placenta is a dangerous distraction interfering with oxytocin release. It is related to the widespread ritual separation of mother and newborn baby. Teaching the whole world that cutting the cord is not a physiological necessity would have enormous public health consequences. Few people know that some hours after the birth the cord is thin, dry, hard, and exsanguine. It can then be cut without any special precaution. One of the effects of transmitting this knowledge would be to eradicate neonatal tetanus, a major cause of neonatal deaths in developing countries.[10] Neonatal tetanus is a consequence of early cord cutting and of unclean umbilical cord care practices. Another effect of making this knowledge more widespread would be to weaken the reasons to routinely facilitate the delivery of the placenta with the use of drugs: these drugs block the release of the main love hormone just after the birth of the baby. In terms of civilisation, making love hormones useful again in such a critical period should be a primary objective.

12

Futuristic strategies

Aiming at a precautionary approach regarding the use of drugs during labour is at first sight entering the world of utopia. Today the number of women who give birth to baby and placenta without any pharmacological assistance is so small that obstetrical strategies inspired by precautionary approaches may be deemed unrealistic. Let us qualify them as futuristic.

Such futuristic strategies will first imply that the basic needs of labouring women have been rediscovered and that many aspects of the current deep-rooted cultural conditioning have been overcome. In other words, they will imply the emergence of a paradigm shift. They will also imply that the recent technical advances that make the caesarean an easy, fast, and safer than ever operation are acknowledged, even among the natural childbirth movements. In the age of plastic catheters these advances include safer techniques in anaesthesiology.

The first step towards new strategies will be to identify and to classify the situations it is better to avoid. We have already listed the many crucial unanswered questions related to the use of drips of synthetic oxytocin. Because of the lack of full scientific certainty, there are good reasons to avoid in particular labours with long hours of drips of oxytocin, often associated with epidural anaesthesia, with the risk of finishing with a forceps, a ventouse, or even a caesarean. There are also good reasons to avoid planned pre-labour caesareans. When a pre-labour caesarean has been scheduled there is no guarantee that the baby – particularly its lungs – is perfectly mature. Maternal and fetal hormones associated with the progress of labour contribute to achieve the maturation of the lungs. The increased risks of respiratory problems are well documented.[1,2] In general a non-labour caesarean implies that the fetus has not participated in the initiation of labour. It also implies that the fetus has not been given the opportunity to put into action its system of stress hormones. Breastfeeding difficulties are more probable than after an in-labour caesarean. Furthermore the chances for a successful vaginal birth after caesarean seem to be better in the case of an in-labour caesarean. Real emergency c-sections should also be avoided as much as possible, that is when there is a race between the surgeon and the progress of a fetal distress. These hasty operations are often performed in bad technical conditions and are associated with comparatively poor outcomes.

Finally we must start to prepare for a binary strategy, with two basic scenarios.

In the first scenario the first stage is straightforward by the vaginal route. In this case the point is just to avoid useless interferences.[3] The second scenario is where the birth process is difficult. In this case, in the context of the twenty-first century, it is often better not to procrastinate and the best alternative may be an 'in-labour non-emergency' caesarean. Babies born in such situations are more often than not in very good shape. In this framework we can include 'planned in-labour' c-sections. This is when a c-section has been decided, but it has also been decided to wait until the spontaneous initiation of labour to do the operation.

With such a simplified binary strategy, the point is to decide early enough during the first stage of labour when a caesarean is indicated. We need new tests adapted to twenty-first century strategies. These tests can also often be presented as non-pharmacological ways to try to overcome difficult phases of labour before deciding on the c-section.

13

Interpreting labour pain

When pain appears to be the main obstacle to the progress of labour – a well-known situation – effective non-pharmacological methods of pain relief may be presented as tests adapted to what we call futuristic strategies. They can help to decide at an early stage when the vaginal route is too risky. Their functions will be more easily understood after an overview of the current interpretations of labour pain.

A paradigm shift

Until the scientific advances of the 1970s, the dominant theories were assuming that the pain in labour is not physiological. It was either interpreted in the framework of conditional reflexes (the point of view of the Pavlovian schools of physiology) or considered cultural, particularly among anthropological and psychoanalytical circles. Within these theoretical frameworks, it was as if the pain could be eliminated while the rest of the physiological processes would be maintained. Today we are in a position to understand that there is a physiological pain during labour, but that there is also a physiological system of protection against pain. The important point is that the components of the physiological system of protection against pain have several roles to play, beside pain relief. In other words the pain is part and parcel of the physiological processes.

We have known since the late 1970s that mammals in general and women in particular control the pain of labour by releasing morphine-like substances commonly called endorphins.[1,2] This release of endorphins is one of the components of the physiological system of protection against pain. We learned at the same period that these endorphins (beta-endorphins) stimulate the secretion of prolactin, the motherhood hormone and the key hormone of lactation.[3] It is therefore possible today to interpret a chain of events, which starts with the physiological pain of labour and leads to the release of a hormone considered necessary for the secretion of milk. Any attempt to eliminate electively the pain will neutralise the whole chain of events.

A reduction of the activity of the neocortex is another component of this protective system. When the neocortex is at rest the pain is not integrated into the central nervous system in the same way as in other situations. This is how we can explain the case of women screaming 'it hurts' while being 'on another planet'. In the following days they claim that the birth was not painful.

The depression of memory has obvious protective effects. It is the effect of a reduced neocortical activity, and also of the well-known properties of opiates in general, and therefore of endorphins. The amnesiac effect of oxytocin has also been demonstrated among humans, through experiments confirming the results of animal studies: memory tests have been used after a single dose of intranasal oxytocin.[4]

After such a paradigm shift, the primary objective should not be to make the births painless. The primary objective should be to make the births as easy as possible, so that the need for pharmacological assistance is reduced. When a birth is fast and easy it implies that the hormonal balance is appropriate and that the pain is controlled by the physiological protective system. Finally, once more, we come to the conclusion that the basic needs of labouring women must be rediscovered.

Meanwhile

Meanwhile most modern women have difficult births, including many of those who had planned to stay at home. The pain can reach a pathological degree with such high levels of stress hormones, particularly adrenaline, that the pain itself is the obstacle to the progress of labour. Today such situations are usually treated by epidural anaesthesia. These epidural anaesthesias are usually effective at breaking a vicious circle, so that the dilation can progress, but they often need to be associated with a drip of synthetic oxytocin and the risks are high to finish with a vaginal operative delivery (ventouse or forceps).

In the 1970s I developed an interest in the particular case of labours associated with lumbar pains, where the already well-advanced dilation cannot progress. I was looking at non-pharmacological ways to break the pathological vicious circle. This is how I introduced in the medical literature the use of intracutaneous injections of sterile water and of birthing pools.

Lumbar reflexotherapy

In 1960 I learned from an old surgeon a spectacular trick to treat acute kidney pains. It was the unilateral intracutaneous injections (one or two papules like nettle stings) of sterile water in the costomuscular angle, which is the depression just below the last rib. The injection is painful but it is a local pain that does not last more than a few seconds. The lumbar pain is eliminated immediately. Only some moderate anterior irradiations tend to persist. Some hours later it might be necessary to repeat the injections. These injections have a diagnostic interest: I found them inefficient in the case of biliary colics, retrocaecal appendicitis and other painful abdominal syndromes.

This is how I thought of using such injections on both sides in obstetrics when cervical dilation does not progress and when the contractions are felt as lumbar pain. I found that when the lumbar pains have gone, only a discomfort above the pubic bone continues while cervical dilation is progressing. Originally I did not dare to write about this empirical method, avoiding the risk of being classified as a magician. The mechanism was too mysterious. I became more audacious when we heard of the 'gate control theory of pain'.[5] This theory could explain how a superficial cutaneous pain could block a painful message originating in a kidney or in the uterus at the level of the spine. It is noticeable that the skin of the costomuscular angle is innervated by the posterior branch of the twelfth dorsal nerve, an appropriate zone, theoretically, to compete with such visceral pains. I was therefore in a position to publish a short paper in a French medical journal about what I decided to call *réflexothérapie lombaire* ('lumbar reflexotherapy').[6]

The diffusion of the technique in non-French-speaking countries was possible through word of mouth. The term *réflexothérapie lombaire* was lost in other languages and the place of injections in the lumbar region became vague. However there were countless randomised controlled trials that confirmed the efficacy of this cheap technique. The *American Journal of Obstetrics and Gynecology* published a systematic review of eighteen trials of any type of complementary and alternative therapies for labour pain.[7] All of these prospective, randomised controlled trials involved healthy pregnant women at term, and contained outcome measures of labour pain. They looked at the effects of acupuncture, biofeedback, hypnosis, intracutaneous sterile water injections, massage, and respiratory autogenic training. Intracutaneous water injection was the only method that constantly appeared effective. However I do not think there is a future for lumbar reflexotherapy, because it is too simple and too cheap.

In the future, in the context of simplified binary strategies, lumbar reflexotherapy might be used mostly as a non-pharmacological test before deciding that a caesarean is indicated. When the dilation does not progress, it means that there is probably a major obstacle.

Birthing pools

While the use of intracutaneous sterile water injections was originally an empiric method that was rationalised after the emergence of scientific theories, on the contrary we were first inspired by physiological considerations when introducing the concept of hospital birthing pools in the 1970s.

When the first stage of labour is difficult and very painful, the first objective should be to try to reduce the level of maternal adrenaline, since adrenaline and oxytocin are antagonistic. A simple way to modify the physiological state can occasionally be detected. For example the room is not warm enough, or there is somebody around releasing the contagious stress hormones. We could anticipate that immersion in water at the same temperature as the body should be a way to reach a state of complete relaxation and therefore a way to lower the level of adrenaline. It should be a way to break a vicious circle.

This is how I first bought an inflatable garden paddling pool and we found a space in the maternity unit to install it. This was the beginning of the history of birthing pools in hospitals.

In 1983 I could already summarise in a mainstream medical journal what it is important to understand and to transmit about the use of birthing pools during labour:[8]

'We tend to reserve the pool for women who are experiencing especially painful contractions (lumbar pain, in particular), and where the dilatation of the cervix is not progressing beyond about 5 cm. In these circumstances, there is commonly a strong demand for drugs. In most cases, the cervix becomes fully dilated within 1 or 2 hours of immersion...' At that time I could only refer to 'most cases'. Afterwards, I analysed the outcomes in the rare cases when the dilation had not progressed after an hour or two in the bath. I finally realised that a caesarean had always been necessary, more often than not after long and difficult first and second stages. This is how I started to tacitly take into account what I had not yet called the birthing pool test.

Recently, at a time when we need to reconsider the usual obstetrical strategies, significant anecdotes encouraged me to give more importance to the birthing pool test. These are two examples of such anecdotes. A woman in hard labour arrived in a maternity unit with her doula while the dilation of the cervix was already well advanced. Soon afterwards this labouring woman entered the birthing pool. More than an hour later the dilation had not progressed although there was an ideal atmosphere of privacy with the lights off. The doula – who was aware of the birthing pool test – was adamant that this woman could not safely give birth by the vaginal route. A senior doctor was eventually called and diagnosed a brow presentation. A brow presentation is difficult to diagnose in early labour and is incompatible with the vaginal route. In this case the doula knew that a caesarean would be necessary, although she could not explain why. The same doula was once with a woman who wanted to try to give birth vaginally after a previous caesarean. At 7 o'clock in the morning, after two hours spent in a birthing pool, the dilation had remained unchanged, around four centimetres. The doula insistently repeated that a caesarean would be necessary. Finally the operation was performed around 12 noon. There was a dehiscence (a 'window') at the level of the uterine scar. The caesarean was undoubtedly necessary.

The birthing pool test is based on the important fact that immersion in water at body temperature tends to facilitate the progress of labour during a limited length of time (in the region of two hours). This simple fact is confirmed by clinical observation and by the results of a Swedish randomised controlled study suggesting that women who enter the bath at 5 cm or after ('late bath group') have a short labour and a reduced need for oxytocin administration and epidural analgesia.[9]

Today we can offer a plausible physiological scenario explaining why immersion in water at body temperature makes the contractions more effective during a limited period of time. When a woman enters the pool in hard labour there is an immediate obvious pain relief, and therefore an immediate reduction in the levels of stress hormones. Since stress hormones and oxytocin are antagonistic, the main short-term response is usually a peak of oxytocin and therefore a spectacular progress in the dilation. After that there is a long-term complex response, which is a redistribution of blood volume. This is the standard response to any sort of water immersion. There is more blood in the chest.[10] When the chest blood volume is increased, certain specialised heart cells in the atria release a sort of hormone commonly called ANP (atrial natriuretic peptide) that interfere with the activity of the posterior pituitary gland.[11] We can all observe the effects of a reduced activity of our posterior pituitary gland after being in a bath for a while: we pass more urine. This means that the release of vasopressin – the water retention hormone – is reduced. In fact the chain of events is not yet completely clarified.[12] We have recently learnt that oxytocin – the love hormone – has receptors in the heart (!) and that it is a regulator of ANP.[13]

In practice we just need to remember that the immediate peak of oxytocin following immersion in warm water will induce a feedback mechanism and eventually the uterine contractions will become less effective after an hour or two.

In general, all the recommendations that should be widely divulged regarding the use of the birthing pool are based on this double response to water immersion.

The first practical recommendation is to give a great importance to the time when the labouring woman enters the pool. Experienced midwives have many tricks at their disposal to help women to be patient enough so that they can ideally wait until the middle of dilation. A shower, which usually implies complete privacy, is an example of what the midwife can suggest while waiting. A survey published in the *British Medical Journal* clearly indicated that many women stay too long in the bath. One reason is that many of them enter the bath long before 5 cm.[14]

The second recommendation is to avoid planning a birth under water. Birth under water is a possibility when it occurs after a short series of irresistible contractions in the pool. It should not become an objective. When a woman has planned a birth under water she may be the prisoner of her project; she is tempted to stay in the bath while the contractions are getting weaker, with the risk of long second and third stages. In general, women should avoid having a precise preconceived script of what the birth of their baby will be like. It is commonplace to wrongly associate 'waterbirth' and 'natural childbirth'. We must keep in mind that seals – highly aquatic mammals – give birth on the dry land. We must also keep in mind that the sense of smell – which is important in the interaction between mother and newborn baby – is neutralised after a birth under water.

Let us add a simple recommendation regarding the temperature. It is easy to check that the water temperature is never above 37°C (the temperature of the maternal body). Two cases of neonatal deaths have been reported after immersion during labour in prolonged hot baths (39.7°C in one case).[15] The proposed interpretation was that the fetuses had reached high temperatures (the temperature of a fetus is 1° higher than the maternal temperature) and could not meet their increased need for oxygen. The fetus has a problem of heat elimination.

At the dawn of a new phase in the history of childbirth one can anticipate that, if a small number of simple recommendations were taken into account, the use of water immersion – in the case of difficult labour – could seriously compete with the use of drugs, particularly synthetic oxytocin and epidural anaesthesia.

In general, the development of non-pharmacological methods of pain relief should be considered as one of the necessary steps towards a precautionary approach regarding pharmacological assistance during labour.

14

The future of pharmacological assistance in childbirth

Until now pharmacological assistance in childbirth has been based on a simplistic principle, which is hormonal replacement. This led to the typical scenario of modern birth, with an intravenous drip of synthetic oxytocin to replace the release of natural oxytocin, and an epidural analgesia, as a substitute for the natural morphine-like substances. Even if, in the near future, the basic needs of labouring women are universally accepted, even if the paradigm shift we are dreaming of is actually emerging, and even if non-pharmacological methods for facilitating the physiological processes develop, one cannot imagine the end of pharmacological assistance in childbirth.

Learning from clinical observation

One can anticipate, however, the development of a new basis for this kind of assistance. This new step will imply that the specifically human handicap in childbirth is understood. In other words, it implies that the concept of neocortical inhibition is not ignored any more.

This leads me to recall how, in 1964, I suddenly and unexpectedly understood the most important aspect of birth physiology. A friend of mine, a medical doctor working for a French pharmaceutical firm, gave me some samples of the recently synthesised gamma-hydroxybutyric acid (GHB). In the context of the 1960s he was already in a position to explain that it was an analogue of GABA (gamma-aminobutyric acid) and that it could not be dangerous since it was an integral part of the mammalian central nervous system.[1] This newly commercialised substance was presented as a sedative medication and as a promising agent in anaesthesiology. My friend added that, according to several preliminary reports, it also shared the properties of oxytocin.

This is how I had the experience of births with drips of what is called in France gamma-OH. With such a drip, labouring women were going completely crazy, shouting in the corridors, pulling out their intravenous needle, scaring the midwife . . . but the baby was born right away. Of course such scenes were unacceptable in a hospital setting and we had to be cautious with possible unreported negative side effects. The main result of this audacious experiment – that we had to stop immediately – was a sort of revelation. I had understood that, when the activity of the neocortex is eliminated, human beings have more similarities with the other mammals: this is what makes birth easy. I had understood the concept of neocortical inhibition and the solution nature had found to overcome the human handicap. The important point was to realise that the neocortex of a labouring woman must not be stimulated.

Since that time we have learned a lot about the inhibitory effects of GHB and GABA.[2] In fact GHB has found limited clinical use as an anaesthetic agent. On the other hand, a widespread interest in this drug developed recently, because it has emerged as a major recreational drug and public health problem. Illicit forms are available under a number of names, such a G, or liquid ecstasy. Its property to neutralise neocortical inhibitions explains the notoriety of this 'date-rape drug' – in other words a compound used to facilitate sexual assault.

My understanding of the effects of neocortical inhibition in childbirth was reactivated about ten years later through another significant anecdote. A young mother was celebrating the birth of her one-day-old baby in a double bedroom. Her neighbour was in pre-labour. This is how glasses of champagne were exchanged. The effect of champagne was so spectacular that a baby was born through a 'fetus ejection reflex' on the way to the birthing room.[3] It is well known that champagne is a special wine. Thanks to the bubbles, alcohol is brought immediately to the brain. The ability of alcohol to change human consciousness has been known for ages. Today we understand how alcohol works: one of its effects is to bind to the GABA receptors.[4]

I also learned a lot from the easy way schizophrenic women were giving birth before the widespread use of powerful antipsychotic treatments. It has been demonstrated that unmedicated schizophrenic people have neocortical inhibition deficits. Interestingly powerful antipsychotic drugs such as clozapine tend to potentiate the effects of GABA.[5]

Learning from word of mouth

It is significant that the psychedelic drugs used for their spiritual virtues have also been used to facilitate labour. This is the case for cannabis, which has been, and still is, a Holy plant in many cultures all over the world. Although some European countries, Canada, and some US states have legalised medical cannabis, it is only through anecdotes and word of mouth that we are learning about its actual effects in the particular case of the birth process. The biochemical effects of the cannabinoids – the most prevalent psychoactive substances in cannabis – have been widely studied. In 1990, the discovery of cannabinoid receptors located throughout the brain and body, along with endogenous cannabinoid neurotransmitters, suggested that cannabis affects the brain in the same manner as a naturally occurring brain chemical. Cannabinoids play an easy to observe role in neocortical activity, with a distortion of the perception of time and space; furthermore, they affect pain transmission by interacting with the system of endorphins.[6] Their effects on the birth process can therefore be easily interpreted.

The daime, a drink known generically as ayahuasca, is

another typical example of a drug used for both its spiritual virtues and its reputation to facilitate the birth process. It is the basis of a spiritual practice, the Santo Daime, which was founded in the Brazilian Amazonian state of Acre in the 1930s and became a worldwide movement in the 1990s. Because the daime is legal for religious use in Brazil, some midwives know about the effects of this drug during labour and do not hesitate to report their observations. This decoction is made from two or more plants, such as the leaves of *Psychotria viridis*, which have high concentrations of the psychoactive compound dimethyltryptamine. Not only is this substance found in many plants, but it is also created in small amounts by the human body during normal metabolism. Its natural function remains undetermined. The stomach normally digests it, so that it does not reach the brain if consumed orally, except if it is mixed with a monoamine oxidase inhibitor (MAOI). Interestingly the daime also contains a vine, such as *Banisteriopsis caapi*, which is a source of MAOI. One can wonder how the natives found this combination without knowing anything about the interaction in the stomach of dimethyltryptamine and MAOI!

All drugs have side effects

The point is not to promote the use in childbirth of GHB, marijuana, daime, or even champagne. It is instead to learn from the effects of drugs that do not belong to the official pharmacopoeia, and to realise that as long as birth physiology is not understood as a chapter of brain physiology, pharmacological assistance in childbirth is reduced to hormonal replacement. The current dominant approach is based on the use of substitutes for oxytocin, endorphins, and prostaglandins. It is possible that in the near future a greater importance will be given to the concept of neocortical inhibition. New questions about plastic-related substances such as phthalates, and new questions about the transfer of synthetic oxytocin across the placenta and the fetal blood-brain barrier will justify a more cautious use of what is today the main component of pharmacological assistance in childbirth.

However all drugs have side effects and it takes time to evaluate the risks and benefits of new pharmacological agents. In the case of drugs that interfere with brain functions, it will be essential to think long term, in other words to take into account the primal health research perspective. This is suggested by animal experiments, such as those by Carol Kellogg, who studied the long-term consequences on the offspring of diazepam – a widely used sedative drug acting on the GABA receptors. One of the significant conclusions of her experiments is that exposure to this drug at the end of fetal life induces behavioural effects that do not become apparent in exposed animals until young adult ages.[7] There are other significant conclusions of these series of studies suggesting the need to think long term when manipulating brain receptors during the early phases of development. For example, if male rats have been exposed to diazepam before being born, the expected adolescent surge of testosterone does not occur.[8]

The importance of keeping in mind the possible long-term effects of drugs used during the perinatal period is also a lesson to learn from studies by Bertil Jacobson and Karin Nyberg about the risk factors for drug addiction: opiates and nitrous oxide used during labour appear as risk factors in all their studies.[9,10,11,12]

Finally, even if a more cautious approach regarding pharmacological assistance in obstetrics is probable during the twenty-first century, and even if the concept of in-labour non-emergency caesarean is better understood, the priority will always be to rediscover the basic needs of labouring women, as long as the main objective is to facilitate in our societies the release of an abundant flow of love hormones in critical periods of human life.

15

The industrialisation of pregnancy in the age of cheap plastics

In the age of cheap plastic, all aspects of human activities are more or less industrialised. Industrialisation includes the concept of standardisation.[1] We must realise that modern women reach the term of their pregnancies in an emotional state highly influenced by standardised prenatal care. This issue must be looked at seriously when considering all the possible steps towards a precautionary approach regarding the use of drugs during labour.

Are they still 'normal' pregnant women?

It is well understood that the prerequisite for the labour to establish itself properly is a low level of anxiety. In other words, the more a pregnant woman is subjected to anxiety-provoking stimuli, the more difficult the birth process is bound to be. A low level of anxiety is also the prerequisite for an optimal growth and development of the baby in the womb: important considerations at a time when we have begun to realise that our health is to a great extent shaped in the womb.

The preliminary practical questions must therefore focus on the possible effects of standardised intensive prenatal care on the emotional state of pregnant women.

In our daily life all of us can notice that it has become impossible to meet a 'normal' pregnant woman. All of them have been given at least one reason to be seriously worried. "You are too old or you are too young", "your blood pressure is too high or too low", "according to the blood sample you are at risk of having a Down's syndrome baby", "you did not take folic acid at the right time and we must consider the risk of spina bifida", "you are not immunised against rubella", "you are Rh negative", "your weight is increasing too quickly or too slowly", "you are anaemic: you must correct that with supplements of iron", "you might haemorrhage because your platelet count is low", "you have gestational diabetes", "your baby is too small or too big", "there is too much liquid around the baby", "there is a lack of liquid", "the placenta is low", "we suspect from the last scan that there is a loop of the cord around the baby's neck", "your baby has not yet turned head first", "you have B streptococci in your vagina", "in our country we routinely test for toxoplasmosis and cytomegalovirus", "if you have not given birth on Wednesday, we must consider an induction", etc. Finally, when the labour is ready to start, it appears that the baby's back is on the right side: births are easier when the baby's back is on the left side.

It is obvious that the dominant style of prenatal care – constantly focusing on potential problems – has an inherent 'nocebo effect'. The nocebo effect is a negative effect on the emotional state of pregnant women and indirectly of their families. It occurs whenever a health professional does more harm than good by interfering with the imagination, the fantasy life or the beliefs of a patient or a pregnant woman.[1]

Until now the medical establishment tends to ignore the effects of standardised prenatal care on the emotional state of pregnant women. This lack of interest can be illustrated by the contents of a special issue of *The Lancet* dedicated to diabetes, and in particular by the three papers focusing on pregnancy: there is no reference to the power that the term 'gestational diabetes' has to transform a happy pregnant woman into an anxious or depressed one.[2,3,4] I was given the opportunity to comment on these articles.[5] Let us recall that 'gestational diabetes' is the interpretation of a test – the glucose tolerance test – that is routinely offered in many countries: if the peak of glycaemia (amount of glucose in the blood) is considered too high after absorption of sugar, the test is positive. This diagnosis has a limited interest because it merely leads to simple recommendations that should be given to all pregnant women. A huge Canadian study demonstrated that the only effect of routine glucose tolerance screening was to inform about three per cent of pregnant women that they have gestational diabetes.[6] The diagnosis did not change the birth outcomes. In my comments I suggested that, instead of using this term, it might be more cost-effective to routinely spend longer than usual discussing with *all* pregnant women several aspects of their lifestyle, in particular the importance of daily physical activity and, in the age of soft drinks and white bread, issues such as high versus low glycaemic index foods. While the glucose tolerance test was presented in *The Lancet* articles as 'an opportunity of a lifetime' for detecting women at risk of developing a non-insulin-dependent diabetes later on in life, I suggested that it would be better to make antenatal care 'an opportunity of a lifetime' for reconsidering several aspects of our modern lifestyle? Instead of focusing on the prevention of a limited number of maternal disorders, would it not be more advantageous to positively promote health and to develop long-term thinking? In other words I suggested ways to reconsider the dominant style of prenatal care.

Evidence supporting the dominant style of prenatal care

Before suggesting ways to reconsider the dominant style of prenatal care, we must first wonder if the very concept of routine medicalised care with a great number of prenatal visits is supported by evidence. In fact a review of the medical literature suggests that it is based on beliefs rather than scientific data.

British studies failed to find any association between beginning prenatal care late and adverse outcomes for the mother or the baby[7] or between the number of visits and the onset of the disease eclampsia.[8] Within the British National

Health Service, the number of visits is not as strongly associated with socio-economic status as it is in the USA. This makes the results of the British studies comparatively easier to interpret than those of the American studies.[9,10]

However, it is worth analysing a 2002 report by the Centers for Disease Control and Prevention in the USA. It appears that women who were born outside the USA are more likely than their racial and ethnic counterparts born in the USA to begin prenatal care late or to have no prenatal care at all. 'In spite of that' (or perhaps 'because of that'?) state-born women are more likely than their counterparts born outside the United States to give birth preterm or to give birth to a low-weight baby. It is also fruitful to analyse trials comparing different schedules of antenatal visits. One was conducted in California, in a Kaiser Permanente Medical Center.[11] A second trial, in south-east London, involved 2,794 women.[12] A third one, by the World Health Organization, involved 53 centres in Thailand, Cuba, Saudi Arabia and Argentina.[13] None of these trials demonstrated any benefits of conventional schedules compared with reduced visit schedules.

One may also wonder if women who have a great number of antenatal visits give birth more easily than those with none. A study on the effect of cocaine use on the progress of labour unexpectedly suggested the opposite.[14] The researchers took into account that one-third of cocaine users had no prenatal care. It was therefore essential to determine the average dilation at admission among non-users of cocaine who had no prenatal care. It appeared that the mean dilation at admission in this group was more than 5 cm.

A paradigm shift

There are therefore reasons to challenge the very concept of routine medicalised care and to shift towards a selective attitude. A selective attitude, based on an adaptation to every particular case, would imply that the main preoccupation of doctors and other health professionals involved in prenatal care should be to protect the emotional state of pregnant women. It also implies that the expectant mother would be guided by a primary practical question: "What can the doctor do for me and my baby?" If we consider the usual case of a woman who knows that she is pregnant, who knows when her baby was conceived, and who is not complaining about anything, the humble response should be: "Not a lot, apart from detecting a gross abnormality and offering an abortion".

Hard data, published in authoritative medical journals, might hasten what would be a real paradigm shift. A typical example is provided by studies of ultrasound scanning. Routine ultrasound scanning in pregnancy became the symbol of modern prenatal care. It is its most expensive component. It often has a nocebo effect. A series of studies compared the effects on birth outcomes of routine ultrasound screening versus the selective use of the scans. An American trial involved more than 15,000 pregnant women.[15] The last sentence of the article is unequivocal: "The findings of this study clearly indicate that ultrasound screening does not improve perinatal outcome in current US practice". Around the same time, an article in the *British Medical Journal*[16] assembled data from four other comparable trials. The authors concluded: "Routine ultrasound scanning does not improve the outcome of pregnancy in terms of an increased number of live births or of reduced perinatal morbidity. Routine ultrasound scanning may be effective and useful as a screening for malformation. Its use for this purpose, however, should be made explicit and take into account the risk of false positive diagnosis in addition to ethical issues". We have already mentioned how useful non-scheduled ultrasound scans can be, particularly in the case of prolonged pregnancies, when the baby might be overdue.

It is possible that, in the future, a new generation of studies (in the framework of primal health research) will cast doubts on the absolute safety of repeated exposure to ultrasound during fetal life. One of the effects of the selective use is to reduce dramatically the number of scans, particularly in the vulnerable phase of early pregnancy.

Even in a high-risk population of pregnant women, ultrasound scans are not as useful as commonly believed. Evidence from several trials suggests that sonographic identification of fetal growth retardation does not improve outcome despite increased medical surveillance.[17,18] In diabetic pregnancies it has been demonstrated that ultrasound measurements are not more accurate than clinical examination to identify high-birthweight babies.[19] This led to the memorable title of an editorial in the *British Journal of Obstetrics and Gynaecology*: 'Guess the weight of the baby'.

Published hard data should also lead to a reconsideration of the measure of haemoglobin concentration in pregnancy. There is a widespread belief that this test can effectively detect anaemia and iron deficiency. In fact, it cannot diagnose iron deficiency because the blood volume of pregnant women is supposed to increase dramatically, so the haemoglobin concentration indicates first the degree of blood dilution, an effect of placental activity. A large British study, involving more than 150,000 pregnancies,[20] found that the highest average birthweight was in the group of women who had a haemoglobin concentration between 8.5 and 9.5. Furthermore, when the haemoglobin concentration fails to fall below 10.5 there is an increased risk of low birthweight and preterm birth. The regrettable consequence of routine evaluation of haemoglobin concentration is that, all over the world, millions of pregnant women are wrongly told that they are anaemic and are given iron supplements. There is a tendency both to overlook the side effects of iron (constipation, diarrhoea, heartburn, etc.) and to forget that iron inhibits the absorption of such an important growth factor as zinc.[21] Furthermore, iron is an oxidative substance that can exacerbate the production of free radicals and might even increase the risk of pre-eclampsia.[22]

Even the routine measurement of blood pressure in pregnancy may be reconsidered. Its original purpose was to detect the preliminary signs of pre-eclampsia, particularly at the end of a first pregnancy. But increased blood pressure, without any protein in the urine, is associated with good birth outcomes.[23,24,25,26] The prerequisite to diagnose pre-eclampsia is the presence of more than 300 mg of protein in the urine per twenty-four hours. Finally, it is more useful to rely on the repeated use of the special strips for 'urinalysis' one can buy in any pharmacy. Measuring the blood pressure is thus not essential.

From knowledge to awareness

By presenting an overview of what we know and what we do not know, one of our objectives has been to justify a precautionary approach regarding the use of drugs, particularly synthetic oxytocin, during labour. Our objective has also been to underline that such a new approach implies a shift towards radically new attitudes and strategies. It implies more than knowledge: knowledge must be digested. In other words it would be based on the emergence of a new awareness. New awareness is not a matter for specialised health professionals only. It should involve the general public – particularly pregnant women – and therefore the media.

We must also constantly keep in mind that all aspects of our lifestyle, including the way babies are born, can be highly influenced by unexpected spectacular technical advances. This is the lesson we can learn from the history of plastic.

16

Clarified objectives

Today plastics are so ubiquitous that we barely notice them. They are the primary determinants of most aspects of our modern lifestyle. For example, it is commonplace to refer to the twenty-first century as the information age. We must keep in mind that plastic computer discs and audio- and videotapes are the basis of information technology.

In such a context the point is not to prepare for a post-plastic age, particularly in medicine. We can only clarify what our ultimate objectives should be whatever the nature of the spectacular technical advances that will emerge at a probably breathtaking speed during the next decades. These objectives appear unrealistic when expressed in the usual way, which is a negative way: reducing the rates of caesareans, avoiding the use of synthetic oxytocin and other obstetrical interventions. They become more easily understood, accepted, and even realistic when expressed in a positive way:

The primary objective of the twenty-first-century generations should be to learn to create the situations where as many women as possible on this planet can give birth to babies and placentas thanks to the release of cocktails of love hormones.

Can the current global financial pre-occupations and the possible shift towards negative economical growth be the driving force towards a sudden new salutary awareness?

Let us parody a comment by Albert Einstein on the release of atomic energy. The plastic revolution has not created a new problem: it has merely made more urgent the necessity of solving existing ones.

17

The cost of childbirth in the age of plastics

Cost-effectiveness is the main reason why most human activities became gradually more industrialised and therefore centralised and standardised, be it the breeding of chickens, the distribution of food in supermarkets, or the check-in process in airports. There is a positive correlation between cost-effectiveness and degree of industrialisation.

What is Earth Overshoot Day?

At a time when humanity is in a position of debtor, it is obvious that we must urgently find solutions to moderate health expenses in general, and expenses related to childbirth in particular. Today, the independent think tank Global Footprint Network[*] provides some of the best tools to explain the alarming situation in which humanity finds itself. The goal of this authoritative network is to create a future where all humans can live well, within the means of one planet Earth. Its concept of Ecological Debt Day, or Earth Overshoot Day, is an eloquent way to convince anyone that humanity is as if overdrawn. Earth Overshoot Day is the day in a year by which humanity has consumed as many of Earth's ecological services as nature can provide in a whole year. The first Earth Overshoot Day was December 19, 1987. In 2009, it occurred on September 25. In 2010, on August 21st. In all developed countries the growth of health expenses is faster than economic growth, and has reached such a point that, in the USA, the total spending on health is already 16% of the enormous American gross domestic product (GDP). The plastic revolution has contributed to

---

[*] www.footprintnetwork.org

the creation of an an overtreated society.

Since the beginning of the history of plastics and until now – the period we have studied – the history of childbirth has been mostly influenced by technical advances. It is becoming clear that from now on, economic factors will prevail upon all the others. This is one way among others to repeat that the history of childbirth is at a turning point. Within the next decades two groups of possible scenarios are plausible, leading the history of childbirth towards two possible opposite directions.

Two possible scenarios

One of the two plausible scenarios is a confirmed tendency towards a still higher degree of industrialisation, which implies a higher degree of centralisation and standardisation. This tendency is very probable in the near future with the development of e-health. It is plausible, for example, that the body of more and more pregnant women will carry a tiny device – a chip – that will transmit to a centralised office the fluctuations of biological parameters such as glycaemia. The cost-effectiveness of such practices will not be easily evaluated, since it will have to take into account the expected interferences with the emotional states of the carriers of such devices. We can already observe this ubiquitous tendency towards a higher degree of industrialisation for the birth itself: closing small maternity units and merging others.

From a short-term perspective this gradual evolution will probably have the support of most decision-makers familiar with the rules of economics. It already has the tacit support of many associations of obstetricians. The ultimate step would be, in huge departments of obstetrics, to perform dozens of elective c-sections every weekday from 9 am to 5 pm. It would be easy to demonstrate how cost-effective this caricature of industrialised obstetrics is, and how safe it is if perinatal mortality and morbidity rates, plus maternal mortality and morbidity rates, are the only criteria taken into account.

Of course such extreme degrees of industrialised obstetrics will be an easy-to-explain threat for the future of humanity, since it will imply the uselessness of love hormones in the critical periods surrounding birth. This is why it should induce, one day or another, a sudden new awareness. The main questions are about the timing of the circumstances that might induce such a necessary turning point. If it occurs in the near future, before a point of no return, one can imagine, in order to control the cost of childbirth, scenarios based on the fact that even today, although obstetrics in general is extremely expensive, some births remain cheap: there are still women giving birth without any kind of medical intervention, with only the presence of a midwife. Economic considerations, combined with a new awareness related to the uselessness of love hormones, might be a point of departure for a real paradigm shift.

Flirting with Utopia

Such alternative scenarios will become realistic on the day when the basic needs of labouring women are rediscovered. This is why it is so urgent to digest crucial physiological concepts such as the concepts of adrenaline-oxytocin antagonism and the concepts of neocortical inhibition. Then the art of midwifery will be understood as the art of creating the conditions for real 'fetus ejection reflexes'. Is the physiological perspective strong enough to reverse the effects of a deep-rooted conditioning? Rediscovering the basic needs of labouring women would lead to radically reconsider the relationship between midwifery and obstetrics, including the ratio between the number of obstetricians and the number of midwives. It would also lead to a reconsideration of the way midwives and obstetricians are selected and trained. Can we imagine that to be a midwife or an obstetrician the prerequisite is to be a mother who has given birth with her own physiological means? One cannot consider the future of humanity without flirting with utopia.

Trying to reduce the cost of childbirth by making the births as easy as possible would also imply a renewed importance given to the emotional states of pregnant women. It is difficult to evaluate the indirect cost of alterations of maternal emotional states induced by the dominant style of routine prenatal care. It is probably enormous since the widespread iatrogenic anxiety is undoubtedly a factor influencing fetal growth and fetal development, and also a factor explaining the difficulties modern women have in giving birth in hospitals and at home. Creating such situations that most women could spend their pregnancy with a level of anxiety as low as possible would be a paradoxically unfamiliar, even futuristic, objective in obstetrics.

An appropriate analysis of valuable studies published in the authoritative medical literature would be a significant step in reducing the cost of pregnancy. Since ultrasound scans are an important part of these expenses, the studies demonstrating that routine ultrasound screening does not improve perinatal outcome, compared with only ultrasound scans on demand, should be rescued from oblivion and discussed.[1,2]

Other routine pregnancy tests might inspire similar comments. This is the case for the glucose tolerance test, leading to the term 'gestational diabetes', which has the power to transform a happy pregnant woman into an anxious or depressed one overnight. The study regarding the regions of Canada where routine glucose tolerance tests have been abandoned should also be rescued from oblivion, since the perinatal outcomes were ultimately the same as elsewhere.[3] It is not surprising that more and more pregnant women are given the diagnosis of gestational diabetes, at a time when there is an increasing prevalence of obesity and glucose intolerance in the general population. However this term, associated with a strong nocebo effect, is considered useless by the practitioners who take the time to talk in depth with all pregnant women about different aspects of lifestyle, particularly nutrition and physical activity. Generalised health promotion is probably more cost-effective than the detection through sophisticated tests of women more at risk than others of particular pathological disorders.

Meanwhile, in spite of published scientific data, and in spite of economical considerations, it is probable that in the near future the diagnosis of gestational diabetes will still be more common. One of the reasons is the tendency to modify the current thresholds for the diagnosis of gestational diabetes. The expected effects of the new criteria proposed by the authoritative International Association of Diabetes and Pregnancy Study Groups (IADPSG) will be to double the number of women diagnosed with gestational diabetes, and to increase the burden on high-risk maternity care.[4] These new attitudes are based on the interpretation of studies comparing non-treated and treated cases of gestational diabetes.[5,6,7] The main flaw shared by all these studies is that in the so-called treated group they include and mix dietary advice (without any detail) and injections of insulin 'if needed'. Recommendations about daily physical activity are never mentioned. Finally, although the only demonstrated effects of 'treatment' is to restrict fetal growth (including brain growth), most practitioners conclude and transmit the idea that gestational diabetes is a disease they must treat.

We took the example of the glucose tolerance test and gestational diabetes to suggest the urgent need to reconsider the dominant way of medical thinking in general. Today the focus is on the prevention and the treatment of specific pathological disorders. Can economic considerations become the driving force able to induce a shift towards a new way of thinking dominated by the concept of health promotion?

We might extend our questions to other fields of medicine. The reason why modern medicine is responsible for an uncontrolled waste of money is related to the dominant medical way of thinking, exclusively focusing on the treatment of pathological conditions. A whole generation of health professionals, particularly doctors, has never been taught the value of therapeutic abstention or minimal intervention, even in the most common pathological situations. For example I know of several young school children whose broken forearm has been treated by osteosynthesis (treating a fracture with implantable devices such as metal plates, pins, rods and screws), while surgeons my generation know that an approximate reduction of the displaced bones followed by immobilisation in plaster would be the guarantee of a perfect functional and aesthetic result, at a low cost and without any risk.

The dominant way of thinking is reinforced by the lack of experience of many practitioners. Inexperienced doctors are expensive. At a time when it is commonplace to complain about the shortage of obstetricians and midwives, it is provocative to mention, on the contrary, their overabundance, and therefore the lack of experience of most of them. There are objective ways to evaluate this overabundance. For example, in the USA, the number of obstetricians is in the region of 40,000. The number of births a year is in the region of four million. This means that a typical American obstetrician is in charge of about 100 births a year: a dangerous lack of experience. During many years I have been the only doctor in charge of 1,000 births a year. I thought at that time that it was a minimum to maintain a valuable level of experience.

Is a dramatic reduction of medical doctors a solution to reduce a part of the debt humanity has towards Mother Earth? Undoubtedly this solution will be currently deemed utopian.

Is it also utopian to establish radically new criteria to select those who will become obstetricians or midwives, the prerequisite being to be a mother who has had the experience of birthing without medical intervention?

Is it utopian to rediscover what a birth can be when

there is nobody around the labouring woman, apart from an experienced and silent midwife perceived as a mother figure?

More generally speaking: is it utopian to control health expenses?

Is it utopian to postpone the Earth Overshoot Day?

Finally, if all the possible solutions are utopian, let us jump to the ultimate question.

Is the survival of humanity utopian?

EPILOGUE

"Problems cannot be solved by the same level of thinking that created them."

Albert Einstein

By studying the industrialisation of childbirth in relation to the plastic revolution, we have realised the limits of the realistic level of thinking and the nature of the problems humanity has to solve urgently. This led us to introduce the concept of utopia and to suggest a necessary combination of utopian and realistic ways of thinking. This is a reason for exploring 'Childbirth in the land of Utopia'.

CHILDBIRTH IN THE LAND OF UTOPIA
JANUARY 2031

As everybody knows, our country – Utopia – is an independent territory.

In spite of our high scientific and technological level, we have maintained and even developed our main cultural characteristics. We have developed in particular our capacity to make unrealistic projects and to smash the limits of political correctness. We shall illustrate the specificity of the Utopian culture by referring to the history of childbirth.

In 2010 two local celebrities had chosen to give birth by caesarean. This is how childbirth suddenly became one of the main topics for discussion in the media. We all realised that every year the rate of caesareans was higher than the year before. The dominant opinion was in favour of authoritarian guidelines by the Utopian Health Organisation (UHO). To face such an unprecedented situation the Head of UHO decided to organise a multidisciplinary meeting.

A statistician spoke first. He presented impressive graphs, starting in 1950, when the low segmental technique of caesarean replaced the classical technique. According to his extrapolations it was highly probable that after 2020 the caesarean would be the most common way to give birth. A well-known obstetrician felt obliged to immediately comment on these data. He claimed that we should look at the positive aspect of this new phenomenon. He explained how the caesarean had become an easy, fast and safe operation. He was convinced that in the near future most women would prefer to avoid the risks associated with a delivery by the vaginal route. To support his point of view about the safety of the caesarean, he presented a Canadian series, published in 2007, of more than 46,000 elective caesareans for breech presentation at 39 weeks with zero maternal death, and an American series, published in 2009, of 24,000 repeated caesareans with one neonatal death. He explained that in many situations an elective pre-labour caesarean was by far the safest way to have a baby. He concluded that 'we cannot stop progress'. While he was speaking the body language of one midwife suggested that there was something the doctor had not understood.

A very articulate lady, the president of BWL (Association for Birth With Love) immediately reacted to the conclusion by the doctor. She first asked him which criteria he was using to evaluate the safety of the caesarean. Of course he just mentioned perinatal mortality/morbidity rates and maternal mortality/morbidity rates. Then the president of BWL explained that this limited list of criteria had been established long ago, before the twenty-first century, and that a great diversity of developing scientific disciplines was now suggesting a list of new criteria to evaluate the practices of obstetrics and midwifery. This was the turning point of this historical multidisciplinary meeting.

The professor of hormonology immediately echoed this

eloquent and convincing comment. After referring to an accumulation of data regarding the behavioural effects of hormones involved in childbirth, he could easily conclude that to have babies women had been programmed to release a real 'cocktail of love hormones'. He clearly explained that during the hour following birth maternal and fetal hormones released during the birth process are not yet eliminated and each of them has a specific role to play in the interaction between mother and neonate. In other words, he added, thanks to the hormonal perspective we can now interpret the concept of critical periods introduced by behavioural scientists: some pioneers in this field had understood, as early as the middle of the twentieth century, that among all mammals there is, immediately after birth, a short period of time that will never happen again and that it is critical in mother-baby attachment. He dared to conclude that by combining the data he had provided with the result of countless epidemiological studies suggesting that the way we are born has life-long consequences it was becoming clear that the capacity to love develops to a great extent in the perinatal period. The obstetrician was gaping at him.

After such conclusions by the professor of hormonology, the head of the department of epidemiology of UHO could not remain silent. This epidemiologist had a special interest in 'Primal Health Research'. He had collected in particular hundreds of published studies detecting risks factors in the perinatal period for a great diversity of pathological conditions in adulthood, adolescence or childhood. He offered an overview of the most valuable studies, particularly those involving huge number of subjects. He summarised the results of his enquiries by noticing that when researchers study, from a Primal Health Research perspective, pathological conditions that can be interpreted as different sorts of impaired capacity to love (to love others or to love oneself), they always detect risk factors in the perinatal period. Referring to the comments by the president of BWL about the needs for new criteria to evaluate the practices of obstetrics and midwifery, he emphasised the need to think long term. Finally he presented the Primal Health Research Databank as a tool to train ourselves to think long term.

Then a geneticist impatiently raised her hand. She presented the concept of 'gene expression' as another way to interpret the life-long consequences of pre- and perinatal events. She explained that among the genetic material human beings receive at conception, some genes will become silent without disappearing. The gene expression phenomenon is influenced in particular by environmental factors during the pre- and perinatal periods. The obstetrician was more and more attentive and curious, as if discovering a new topic. One of his judicious questions about the genesis of pathological conditions and personality traits gave the geneticist the opportunity to explain that the nature of an environmental factor is often less important than the time of the interaction. He explained the concept of critical period for gene-environment interaction. The presentation by the geneticist induced a fruitful interdisciplinary conversation. The epidemiologist jumped on a question by a general practitioner to provide more details about one of the new functions of the Primal Health Research Database, which is to give some clues about the critical period for gene-environment interaction regarding different pathological conditions or personality traits.

A bacteriologist, who had kept a low profile since the beginning of the session, emphasised that the minutes following birth are critical from his perspective as well. Few people had previously understood that at the very time of birth the newborn baby is germ free and that some hours later millions of microbes will have colonised its body. Because the antibodies called IgG easily cross the human placenta he explained that the microbes familiar for the mother are already familiar for the germ-free newborn baby, and therefore friendly. If the baby is immediately contaminated by friendly germs carried by the mother, it is protected against unfamiliar and therefore potentially dangerous microbes. He commented that when babies are born via the perineum, it is a guarantee that they are first contaminated by a multitude of germ satellites of the mother, compared with babies born by caesarean. In order to stress the importance of the question, he mentioned that our gut flora is to a great extent established during the minutes following birth: useful considerations at a time when we are learning that this intestinal flora represents 80% of our immune system.

The bacteriologist agreed when a baby feeding adviser added that, in the right environment, if mother and newborn baby are not separated at all, there is a high probability that the baby will find the breast during the hour following birth and will consume the early colostrum with its friendly germs, specific local antibodies and anti-infectious substances. The consumption of early colostrum probably has long-term consequences, at least by influencing the way the gut flora is established.

The head of UIIO was obviously happy with the progress of the interdisciplinary meeting he had organised. He asked an old philosopher, considered the wise man of the community, to conclude. The philosopher explained that we should not ignore a specifically human dimension and that we must first and foremost think in terms of civilisation. He referred to the data provided by the epidemiologist. Among the studies he presented huge numbers had often been necessary to detect tendencies and statistically significant effects. A way to keep in mind that where human beings are concerned we must often forget individuals, anecdotes and particular cases, and reach the collective and therefore cultural dimension. From what had been heard during this meeting, it was clear that humanity was in an unprecedented situation that he summarised in a very concise way. Today, he said, the number of women who give birth to babies and placentas thanks to the release of what is a real cocktail of love hormones is approaching zero. What will happen in terms of civilisation if we go on that way? What will happen after two or three generations if love hormones are made useless during the critical period surrounding birth?

After such an eloquent conclusion the head of the UHO asked the participants their point of view about the necessity to control the rates of caesarean. Everybody, including the obstetrician, found the need for action necessary, even urgent.

This is how a second meeting was planned in order to find effective solutions.

* * *

At the beginning of the second meeting the head of UHO asked the participants if they had solutions to suggest in order to control the rates of caesareans and other obstetrical interventions. The obstetrician presented a project 'to assess the effectiveness of a multifaceted strategy for improving the appropriateness of indications for caesarean'. Nobody paid attention. A recently graduated young doctor spoke about the need to reconsider the education of medical and midwifery students. The head of the midwifery school immediately replied that all over the world there have been many attempts to re-adapt the education of midwives and doctors, including specialised doctors, without any significant positive effects on birth outcomes. Several participants spoke about financial incentives to moderate the rates of obstetrical intervention. The head of UHO intervened and stressed that this solution had been unsuccessfully tried in several countries and that the rates of c-sections were increasing in all countries whatever the health system: we should therefore look at other factors. He added that the risk would be to increase the incidence of long and difficult births by the vaginal route with an overuse of pharmacological substitutes for the natural hormones. This effect would be unacceptable at a time when the c-section has become such an easy and fast operation. The priority should be to try first to make the births as easy as possible in order to reduce the need for obstetrical interventions in general.

Unexpectedly, the turning point in the discussion occurred when a neurophysiologist – internationally known for her studies of the behaviour of *Mantis religiosa*, a variety of praying mantis – intervened for the first time. She explained that by mixing her scientific studies and her experience as a mother, she had acquired a clear understanding of the basic needs of labouring women. In general, she said, the messages sent by the central nervous system to the genitalia are inhibitory. She understood this simple rule when studying the mating behaviour of *Mantis religiosa*. During sexual intercourse in this species the female often eats the head of the male, a radical way to eliminate inhibitory messages! Then the sexual activity of the male is dramatically reinforced and the chances for offspring conception are increased. She had understood that the inhibitory effect of the central nervous system on all episodes of sexual life is a general rule. She had many occasions to confirm this rule and, interestingly, she understood that still more clearly after giving birth to her first baby. She is convinced that the reduction of her neocortical activity was the main reason why this birth was so easy and fast. She recalled that human beings are characterised by the enormous development of this part of the central nervous system called the neocortex. Her neocortex was obviously at complete rest when she was in established labour since she had completely forgotten many details about the place where she gave birth. She remembers vaguely that she was in a rather dark place, and that there was nobody around but a midwife sitting in a corner and knitting. She also remembers that at a certain phase of labour she was vomiting and the midwife just said: 'this happened to me when I had my second baby: it's normal'. Although this is imprecise in her memory, she is convinced that this discreet comment with a whispering motherly voice had facilitated the progress of labour. With this experienced and calm mother figure she could feel perfectly secure. She can understand in retrospect that all the conditions were met to reduce the activity of her neocortex. She could feel secure without feeling observed, in semi-darkness and silence. So, her practical suggestion, after combining what she learned as a neurophysiologist and what she learned as a mother, was to reconsider the criteria used to select the midwifery students. The prerequisite, to enter a midwifery school of the future, would be to have a personal experience of giving birth without any medical intervention and to consider this birth as a positive experience.

The obstetrician was not comfortable with this suggestion, claiming that he had been working with wonderful midwives who were not mothers. The head of the midwifery school retorted that everybody knows good midwives who are not mothers. However her duty is to offer the guarantee that the midwives graduated in her school share such personality traits that their presence close to a birthing woman will disturb the progress of labour as little as possible. This is why she cannot imagine better criteria than those suggested by the neurophysiologist. Because this suggestion was outside the usual limits of political correctness, it was immediately considered by almost everybody as acceptable in the land of Utopia.

Then a male voice was heard from a corner of the room. It was the voice of the young technician whose role was to record the session: 'as an outsider, can I ask a naïve question? What if the prerequisite to be qualified as an obstetrician would also be to have a personal experience of giving birth without any medical intervention and to consider this birth as a positive experience?'

At that time it was as if everybody in the room was in the situation of Archimedes shouting 'Eureka!' . . . An unforgettable collective enthusiasm! It was immediately obvious for all the participants that such a project was unrealistic enough to be adopted without any further discussion and without any delay in the land of Utopia.

A committee was immediately set up, in order to organise a fifteen-year period of transition.

* * *

Today, in January 2031, we can offer valuable statistics, since the period of transition was over in 2024. These statistics are impressive.

The perinatal mortality rates are as low as in all countries with similar standards of living. The rates of transfers to paediatric units have dramatically decreased. There has not been one case of forceps delivery for four years. Since the priority is to avoid long and difficult labours by the vaginal route, the use of ventouse and the use of drugs are exceptionally rare. However the rates of caesareans are three times lower than before the period of transition. A paedopsychiatrist has already mentioned that autism is less common than in the past. If the respected philosopher – the wise man of the community – was still alive, he would state that now, in the land of Utopia, most women give birth to babies and placentas thanks to the release of a 'cocktail of love hormones'.

The new head of UHO and his teams are preparing articles for different sorts of international media. They have launched a 'call for 5-words slogans' in order to urgently spread the word in a concise and effective way. This is the selected slogan:

ONLY UTOPIA CAN SAVE HUMANITY!

REFERENCES

Chapter 2

1. Mendiola J, Grylack LJ, Scanlon JW. Effects of intrapartum maternal glucose infusion on the normal fetus and newborn. *Anesth Analg* 1982 Jan;61(1):32-5.
2. Lucas A, Adrian TE, Aynsley-Green A, Bloom SR. Iatrogenic hyperinsulinism at birth. *Lancet* 1980 Jan 19;1(8160):144-5.
3. Kenepp NB, Kumar S, Shelley WC, Stanley CA, Gabbe SG, Gutsche BB. Fetal and neonatal hazards of maternal hydration with 5% dextrose before caesarean section. *Lancet* 1982 May 22;1(8282):1150-2.
4. Carmen S. Neonatal hypoglycemia in response to maternal glucose infusion before delivery. *J Obstet Gynecol Neonatal Nurs.* 1986 Jul-Aug;15(4):319-23.
5. Grylack LJ, Chu SS, Scanlon JW. Use of intravenous fluids before cesarean section: effects on perinatal glucose, insulin, and sodium homeostasis. *Obstet Gynecol* 1984 May;63(5):654-8.
6. Kenepp NB, Shelley WC, Kumar S, Gutsche BB, Gabbe S, Delivoria-Papadopoulos M. Effects of newborn of hydration with glucose in patients undergoing caesarean section with regional anaesthesia. *Lancet* 1980 Mar 22;1(8169):645.
7. Singhi S, Sharma S. Neonatal hypoglycemia following maternal glucose infusion prior to delivery. *Indian J Pediatr.* 1991 Jan-Feb;58(1):43-9.
8. Odent M. Laboring women are not marathon runners. *Midwifery Today* Childbirth Educ 1994;(31):23-24,43.
9. Malek A, Blann E, Mattison DR. Human placental transport of oxytocin. *J Matern Fetal Med* 1996 Sep-Oct;5(5):245-55.
10. Saunders NR, Habgood MD, Dziegielewska KM. Barrier mechanisms in the brain, II. immature brain. *Clin Exp Pharmacol Physiol* 1999;26(2):85–91.
11. Braun LD, Cornford EM, Oldendorf WH. Newborn rabbit

blood–brain barrier is selectively permeable and differs substantially from the adult, in *J Neurochem* 1980;34:147–152.

12. Cornford EM, Braun LD, Oldendorf WH. Developmental modulations of blood–brain barrier permeability as an indicator of changing nutritional requirements in the brain, in *Pediatr Res* 1982;16:324–328

13. Brenton DP, Gardiner RM. Transport of L-phenylalanine and related amino acids at the ovine blood–brain barrier, in *J Physiol* 1988;402:497–514.

14. Frank HJ, Jankovic-Vokes T, Pardridge WM, Morris WL. Enhanced insulin binding to blood–brain barrier in vivo and to brain microvessels in vitro in newborn rabbits. In *Diabetes* 1985;34:728–733.

15. Noseworthy M, Bray T. Effect of oxidative stress on brain damage detected by MRI and in vivo 31P-NMR. *Free Rad. Biol Med* 1998;24:942–951.

16. Agnagnostakis D, Messaritakis J, Damianos D, Mandyla H. Blood-brain barrier permeability in healthy infected and stressed neonates. *J Pediatr* 1992;121:291–294.

17. Noseworthy M, Bray T. Zinc deficiency exacerbates loss in blood–brain barrier integrity induced by hyperoxia measured by dynamic MRI. *PSEBM* 2000;231:175–182.

18. Schneid-Kofman N, Silberstein T, Saphier O, Shai I, Tavor D, Burg A. Labor augmentation with oxytocin decreases glutathione level. *Obstet Gynecol Int* 2009:807659. Epub 2009 Apr 16.

19. Robinson C, Schumann R, Zhang P, Young R. Oxytocin-induced desensitization of the oxytocin receptor. *Am J Obstet Gynecol* 2003;188:497–502.

20. Gimpl G, Fahrenholz F. The oxytocin receptor system: structure, function and regulation. *Physiol Rev* 2001;81:642–643.

21. Phaneuf S, Rodríguez Liñares B, TambyRaja RL, MacKenzie IZ, López Bernal A. Loss of myometrial oxytocin receptors during oxytocin-induced and oxytocin-augmented labour. *J Reprod Fertil* 2000 Sep;120(1):91-7.

22. Phaneuf S, Asboth G, Carrasco M, Lineares B, Kimura T, Harris A, et al. Desensitization of oxytocin receptors in human myometrium. *Hum Reprod Update.* 1998;4:625–633.

23. Odent M. *The Scientification of Love*. Free Association Books. London 1999.
24. Modahl C, Green L, et al. Plasma oxytocin levels in autistic children. *Biol Psychiatry* 1998;43(4):270-7.
25. Green L, Fein D, et al. Oxytocin and autistic disorder: alterations in peptides forms. *Biol Psychiatry* 2001;50(8): 609-13.
26. Demitrack MA, Lesem MD, Listwak SJ, et al. CSF oxytocin in anorexia nervosa and bulimia nervosa: clinical and pathophysiologic considerations. *Am J Psychiatry* 1990 Jul;147(7):882-86.
27. Odent M. Autism and anorexia nervosa: two facets of the same disease? *Med Hypotheses* 2010;75(1):79-81. doi:10.1016/j.mehy.2010.01.039.
28. Ming H, Cheng SY, Tsai-Chung L. Titrated oral misoprostol solution compared with intravenous oxytocin for labor augmentation: a randomized controlled trial. *Obst Gynecol* 2010;116(3):612-618. doi:10.1097/AOG.0b013e3181ed36cc.

Chapter 3

1. Lumbiganon P, Laopaiboon M, Gülmezoglu AM, et al. Method of delivery and pregnancy outcomes in Asia: the WHO global survey on maternal and perinatal health 2007-08. *Lancet* 2010 Feb 6;375(9713):490-9. Epub 2010 Jan 11.
2. MacKay DF, Smith GCS, Dobbie R, Pell JP. Gestational age at delivery and special educational need: retrospective cohort study of 407,503 schoolchildren. *PLoS Med* 2010;7(6): e1000289. doi:10.1371/journal.pmed.1000289.
3. Li H-T, Ye R, Achenbach T, Ren A, Pei L, Zheng X, Liu J-M. Caesarean delivery on maternal request and childhood psychopathology: a retrospective cohort study in China. *BJOG* 2010; DOI: 10.1111/j.1471-0528.2010.02762.x.
4. Gitau R, Menson E, Pickles V, et al. Umbilical cortisol levels as an indicator of the fetal stress response to assisted vaginal delivery. *Eur J Obstet Gynecol Reprod Biol* 2001 Sep;98(1):14-7.
5. Mears K, McAuliffe F, Grimes H, Morrison JJ. Fetal cortisol in relation to labour, intrapartum events and mode of delivery. *J*

Obstet Gynaecol 2004;24:129–32.
6. Sørensen HT, Steffensen FH, Sabroe S, et al. Historical cohort study of in utero exposure to uterotonic drugs and cognitive function in young adult life. *West J Med* 1999 May;170(5):260-262.
7. Odent M, Tsufino J. Studies exploring health in relation to intrauterine life should look at birth order. *BMJ* 1997 May 10;314(7091):1416.
8. Seidman DS, Laor A, Gale R, et al. Long term effects of vacuum and forceps deliveries. *Lancet* 1991;337:1583-85.
9. Nilsen ST, et al. Boys born by forceps and vacuum extraction examined at 18 years of age. *Acta Obstet Gynecol Scand* 1984; 63/6:549-554.
10. Hannah ME, Hannah WJ, Hewson SA, et al. Planned caesarean section versus planned vaginal birth for breech presentation at term: a randomised multicentre trial. *Lancet* 2000;256:1375-83.
11. The European Mode of Delivery Collaboration. Elective caesarean-section versus vaginal delivery in prevention of vertical HIV-1 transmission: a randomized clinical trial. *Lancet* 1999; 353:1035-39.
12. Krebs L, Langhoff-Roos J. Elective cesarean delivery for term breech. *Obstet Gynecol* 2003;101(4):690-6
13. Harper MA, Byington RP, Espeland MA, et al. Pregnancy-related death and health care services. *Obstet Gynecol* 2003; 102(2):273-278.
14. Liu S, Liston RM, Joseph KS, et al. Maternal mortality and severe morbidity associated with low-risk planned cesarean delivery versus planned vaginal delivery at term. *CMAJ* 2007;176(4):455-60.
15. Fenton PM, Whitty CJM, Reynolds F. Caesarean section in Malawi: prospective study of early maternal and perinatal mortality. *BMJ* 2003;327:587-90.
16. Pereira C, Bugalho A, et al. A comparative study of caesarean deliveries by assistant medical officers and obstetricians in Mozambique. *Br J Obstet Gynaecol* 1996;103:508-12.

Chapter 4

1. Odent M. *The Scientification of Love.* Free Association Books.

London 1999.

2. Odent M. *Primal Health*. Century Hutchinson. London 1986.

3. Odent M. Attention Deficit Hyperactivity Disorder (ADHD) and obesity: two facets of the same disease? *Med Hypotheses* 2010;74(1):139-141. Epub 2009 Aug 8. doi:10.1016/j. mehy.2009.07.020.

4. Odent M. Autism and anorexia nervosa: two facets of the same disease? *Med Hypotheses* 2010;75(1):79-81. doi:10.1016/j. mehy.2010.01.039.

5. Krehbiel D, Poindron P, et al. Peridural anaesthesia disturbs maternal behaviour in primiparous and multiparous parturient ewes. *Physiol Behav* 1987;40:463-72.

6. Lundbland EG, Hodgen GD. Induction of maternal-infant bonding in rhesus and cynomolgus monkeys after cesarian delivery. *Lab Anim Sci* 1980;30: 913.

7. Hultman C, Sparen P, Cnattingius S. Perinatal risk factors for infantile autism. *Epidemiology* 2002;13:417-23.

8. Odent M. *The Caesarean*. Free Association Books. London 2004.

Chapter 5

1. Gluckman PD, Hanson MA, Cooper C, Thornburg KL. Effect of in utero and early-life conditions on adult health and disease. *NEJM* 2008;359:61-73

2. Kruska D. Mammalian domestication and its effect on the brain structure and behavior. In: *Intelligence and Evolutionary Biology*: 211-250. Jerison I. (eds) Berlin, Eidelberg: Springer 1988.

3. Kruska D. The effect of domestication on brain size and composition in the mink. *J Zool* London 1996;239:645-61.

4. Pembrey ME, Bygren LO, Kaati G, et al. Sex-specific, male-line transgenerational responses in humans. *Eur J Hum Genet* 2006;14:159-66.

5. Ghost in Your Genes, PBS Airdate: October 16 2007, transcript. http://www.pbs.org/wgbh/nova/transcripts/3413_genes.html

6. Kaati G, Bygren LO, Pembrey M, Sjöström M. Transgenerational response to nutrition, early life circumstances and longevity. *Eur J Hum Genet.* 2007

Jul;15(7):784-90. Epub 2007 Apr 25.

7. Pembrey ME. Male-line transgenerational responses in humans. *Hum Fertil* (Camb) 2010 Dec;13(4):268-71.

8. Painter RC, Osmond C, Gluckman P, et al. Transgenerational effects of prenatal exposure to the Dutch famine on neonatal adiposity and health in later life. *BJOG* 2008 Sep;115(10):1243-9.

9. Heijmans BT, Kremer D, Tobi EW, Boomsma DI, Slagboom PE. Heritable rather than age-related environmental and stochastic factors dominate variation in DNA methylation of the human IGF2/H19 locus. *Hum Mol Genet* 2007;16:547-554.

10. Heijmans BT, Tobi EW, Stein AD, et al. Persistent epigenetic differences associated with prenatal exposure to famine in humans. *Proc Natl Acad Sci USA*. 2008;105:17046-49.

11. Van Steijn L, Karamali NS, Kanhai H, et al. Neonatal anthropometry: thin–fat phenotype in fourth to fifth generation South Asian neonates in Surinam. *International Journal of Obesity* 2009(33):1326–9;doi:10.1038/ijo.2009.154; published online 28 July 2009.

12. Varner MW, Fraser AM, Hunter CY, et al. The intergenerational predisposition to operative delivery. *Obstet Gynecol* 1996 Jun;87(6):905-11.

Chapter 6

1. Thurlow JA, Kinsella SM. Intrauterine resuscitation: active management of fetal distress. *Int J Obstet Anesth* 2002;11(2):105-16.

2. Paterson R, Seath J, Taft P. Wood C. Maternal and foetal ketone concentrations in plasma and urine. *Lancet* 1967; ii: 862-5.

3. Johansson S, Lindow S, Kapadia H, Norman M. Perinatal water intoxication due to excessive oral intake during labour. *Acta Paediatr.* 2002;91(7):811-4.

4. Ophir E, Solt I, Odeh M, Bornstein J. Water intoxication - a dangerous condition in labor and delivery rooms. *Obstet Gynecol Surv* 2007 Nov; 62 (II):731-8.

5. Baker RW. Diethylhexyl phthalate as a factor in blood transfusion and haemodialysis. *Toxicology*1978 Apr;9(4):319-29.

6. Cho SC, Bhang SY, Hong YC, et al. Relationship between environmental phthalate exposure and the intelligence of school-aged children. *Environ Health Perspect* 2010 Jul;118(7):1027-32. Epub 2010 Mar 1.

7. Vetrano AM, Laskin DL, Archer F, et al. Inflammatory effects of phthalates in neonatal neutrophils. *Pediatr Res* 2010 Aug;68(2):134-9.

8. Saillenfait AM, Payan JP, Fabry JP, et al. Assessment of the developmental toxicity, metabolism, and placental transfer of Di-n-butyl phthalate administered to pregnant rats. *Toxicol Sci* 1998 Oct;45(2):212-24.

9. Kihlström I, Placental transfer of diethylhexyl phthalate in the guinea-pig placenta perfused in situ. *Acta Pharmacol Toxicol* (Copenh) 1983 Jul;53(1):23-7.

10. Mose T, Knudsen LE, Hedegaard M, et al. Transplacental transfer of monomethyl phthalate and mono(2-ethylhexyl) phthalate in a human placenta perfusion system. *Inter Toxicol* 2007; 26(3):221-9.

11. Balakrishnan B, Henare K, Thorstensen EB, et al. Transfer of bisphenol A across the human placenta. *Am J Obstet Gynecol* 2010;202(4):393.e1-7.

12. Environmental Working Group. *Pollution in People: Cord Blood Contaminants in Minority Newborns.* www.ewg.org/files/2009-Minority-Cord-Blood-Report.pdf.

13. Salian S, Doshi T, Vanage G. Impairment in protein expression profile of testicular steroid receptor coregulators in male rat offspring perinatally exposed to bisphenol A. *Life Sci* 2009;85:11–18.

14. Wu S, Zhu J, Li Y, et al. Dynamic effect of di-2-(ethylhexyl) phthalate on testicular toxicity: epigenetic changes and their impact on gene expression. *Int J Toxicol* 2010 Mar-Apr;29(2):193-200.

15. Habert H, Muczynski A, Lehraiki A, et al. Adverse effects of endocrine disruptors on the fœtal testis development: focus on the phthalates. *Folia Histochem Cytobiol* 2009;47(5):567-74.

16. Kimber I, Dearman RJ. An assessment of the ability of phthalates to influence immune and allergic responses. *Toxicology* 2010 May 27;271(3):73-82. Epub 2010 Apr 3.

17. Wu S, Zhu J, Li Y, et al. Dynamic effect of di-2-(ethylhexyl)

phthalate on testicular toxicity: epigenetic changes and their impact on gene expression. *Int J Toxicol* 2010;29(2):193-200.

18. Yaoi T, Itoh K, Nakamura K, et al. Genome-wide analysis of epigenomic alterations in fetal mouse forebrain after exposure to low doses of bisphenol A. *Biochem Biophys Res Commun.* 2008 Nov 21;376(3):563-7. Epub 2008 Sep 17.

19. Kuruto-Niwa R, Tateoka Y, Usuki Y, Nozawa R. Measurement of bisphenol A concentrations in human colostrums. *Chemosphere* 2007;66(6):1160-4.

Chapter 7

1. Li H-T, Ye R, Achenbach T, Ren A, Pei L, Zheng X, Liu J-M. Caesarean delivery on maternal request and childhood psychopathology: a retrospective cohort study in China. *BJOG* 2011 Jan;118(1):32-8. doi: 10.1111/j.1471-0528.2010.02762.x.

2. Brown VA, et al. The value of antenatal cardiotocography in the management of high-risk pregnancy : a randomised controlled trial. *Br J Obstet Gynaecol* 1982; 89: 716-22.

3. Flynn AM, et al. A randomized controlled trial of non-stress antepartum cardiotocography. *Br J Obstet Gynaecol* 1982;89: 427-33.

4. Lumley JC, Wood C, et al. A randomized trial of weekly cardiotocography in high-risk obstetric patients. *Brit J Obstet Gynaecol* 1983; 90:1018-26.

5. Odent M. Should midwives re-invent the amnioscope? *Midwifery Today Int Midwife* 2006 Winter;(80):7, 66.

6. Michel Odent. *The Caesarean.* Free Association Books. London 2004.

7. Ehrenthal DB, Jiang X, Strobino DM. Labor induction and the risk of a cesarean delivery among nulliparous women at term. *Obstet Gynecol* 2010 Jul;116(1):35-42.

8. Finkel RS, Zarlengo KM. Blue cohosh and perinatal stroke. *N Engl J Med* 2004; 351(3): 302-3.

Chapter 8

1. Odent M. Childbirth in the land of Utopia. *Pract Midwife* 2010 Feb;13(2):4-5.

2. George J, Engelmann. *Labor Among Primitive Peoples.* JH

Chambers & Co. St. Louis 1884.

3. Odent M. Colostrum and civilization. In: Odent M. *The Nature of Birth and Breastfeeding*. Bergin & Garvey 1992. 2nd ed 2003 (*Birth and Breastfeeding*. Clairview).

4. Odent M. Neonatal tetanus. *Lancet* 2008; 371:385-6.

5. Fildes VA. *Breasts, bottles and babies. A history of infant feeding*. Edinburgh University Press, 1986.

6. Klopfer MS, Adams DK. Maternal imprinting in goats. *Proceedings of the National Academy of Sciences* (USA) 1964;52:911-914.

7. Klaus MH, Kennell JH. *Maternal-infant bonding*. CV Mosby. St Louis, 1976.

8. De Chateau P, Wiberg B. Long-term effect on mother-infant behavior of extra contact during the first hour postpartum. I. First observations at 36 hours. *Acta Paediatrica Scand* 1977;66:137.

9. De Chateau P, Wiberg B. Long-term effect on mother-infant behavior of extra contact during the first hour postpartum. II. Follow-up at three months. *Acta Paediatrica Scand* 1977;66:145.

10. Schaller J, Carlsson SG, Larsson K. Effects of extended post-partum mother-child contact on the mother's behavior during nursing. *Infant Behavior and Development* 1979 (2):319-24.

11. Terkel J, Rosenblatt JS. Humoral factors underlying maternal behaviour at parturition: cross transfusion between freely moving rats. *J Comp Physiol Psychol* 1972;80: 365-71.

12. Siegel HI, Greenwald MS. Effects of mother-litter separation on later maternal responsiveness in the hamster. *Physiol Behav* 1978;21:147-9.

13. Siegel HI, Rosenblatt JS. Estrogen-induced maternal behaviour in hysterectomized-ovariectomized virgin rats. *Physiol Behav* 1975 Apr;14(04):465-71.

14. Jeliffe DB, Jeliffe EFP (eds). The uniqueness of human milk. *Am J Clin Nutr* 1971;24:968-1009.

15. Jeliffe DB, Jeliffe EFP. *Human milk in the modern world*. Oxford University Press 1978.

16. McClelland DB, McGrath J, Samson RR. Antimicrobial factors in human milk. Studies of concentration and transfer to the infant during the early stages of lactation. *Acta Paediatr Scand Suppl* 1978;(271):1-20.

17. Odent M. The early expression of the rooting reflex. *Proceedings of the 5th International Congress of Psychosomatic Obstetrics and Gynaecology, Rome 1977*. London: Academic Press, 1977: 1117-19.

18. Odent M. L'expression précoce du réflexe de fouissement. In : *Les Cahiers du Nouveau-Né* 1978;1-2:169-185.

19. Virella G, Silveira Nunes MA, Tamagnini G. Placental transfer of human IgG subclasses. *Clin Exp Immunol* 1972 Mar;10(3):475-8.

20. Pitcher-Wilmott RW, Hindocha P, Wood CB. The placental transfer of IgG subclasses in human pregnancy. *Clin Exp Immunol* 1980 Aug;41(2):303-8.

21. Klaus MH, Kennell JH. *Parent-Infant Bonding*. CV Mosby. St Louis 1982.

Chapter 9

1. Elaine Hatfield, John Cacioppo, Richard Rapson. *Emotional Contagion*. Cambridge University Press. 1993.

2. Odent M. Knitting midwives for drugless childbirth? *Midwifery Today* 2004 Autumn;(71): 21-2.

3. Botvinick, M, Jha, AP, Bylsma, LM, Fabian, SA, Solomon, PE, & Prkachin, KM. Viewing facial expressions of pain engages cortical areas involved in the direct experience of pain. *NeuroImage* 2005;25,312-9.

4. Preston, SD, & de Waal, FBM. Empathy: Its ultimate and proximate bases. *Behavioral and Brain Sciences* 2002;25,1-72.

5. Decety J. Naturaliser l'empathie [Empathy naturalized]. *L'Encéphale* 2002;28,9-20.

6. Decety J, & Jackson, P.L. The functional architecture of human empathy. *Behavioral and Cognitive Neuroscience Reviews* 2044;3,71-100.

Chapter 10

1. Bronislaw Malinowski. *The Sexual Life of Savages*. Horace Liveright 1929.

2. Schiefenhovel W. *Childbirth among the Eipos, New Guinea*. Film presented at the Congress of Ethnomedicine. Gottingen. Germany 1978.

3. Eaton SB, Shostak M, Konner M. *The Paleolithic Prescription.* Harper and Row, New York 1988.
4. Donnison J. *Midwives and Medical Men.* Heinemann, London 1977.
5. Odent M. Knitting midwives for drugless childbirth? *Midwifery Today* 2004; Autumn;(71):21-2.
6. Nissen E, Lilja G, Widström AM, Uvnäs-Moberg K. Elevation of oxytocin levels early post partum in women. *Acta Obstet Gynecol Scand* 1995 Aug;74(7):530-3.
7. Lederman RP, Lederman E, Work BA, McCann DS. Anxiety and epinephrine in multiparous women in labor: relationship to duration of labor and fetal heart rate pattern. *Am J Obstet Gynecol* 1985;153:870-78.
8. Newton N. The fetus ejection reflex revisited. *Birth* 1987;14(2):106-8.
9. Odent M. The fetus ejection reflex. *Birth* 1987;14(2):104-5.
10. Odent M. *The Functions of the Orgasms: the Highways to Transcendence.* Pinter & Martin. London 2009.

Chapter 11

1. Wax et al. Maternal and newborn outcomes in planned home birth vs planned hospital births: a metaanalysis. *Am J Obstet Gynecol* 2010; 203(3):243.el-8.Epub2010Jul2 doi: 10.1016/j.ajog.2010.05.028.
2. Evers AC, Brouwers HA, Hukkelhoven CW, et al. Perinatal mortality and severe morbidity in low and high risk term pregnancies in the Netherlands: prospective cohort study. *BMJ* 2010; 341:c5639. doi: 10.1136/bmj.c5639 (Published 2 November 2010).
3. Peter McDonald. *The Oxford Dictionary of Medical Quotations.* Pers:78. OUP. Oxford 2004.
4. Sosa R, Kennell J, Klaus M, et al. The effect of a supportive companion on perinatal problems, length of labor, and mother-infant interaction. *N Engl J Med* 1980;303:597-600.
5. Klaus M, Kennell J, Robertson SS, Sosa R. Effects of social support on maternal and infant morbidity. *BMJ* 1986;293:585-87.
6. Kennell J, Klaus M, et al. Continuous emotional support during labor in a US hospital. *JAMA* 1991;265:2197-2201.

7. Gordon NP, Walton D, et al. Effects of providing hospital-based doulas in health maintenance organization hospitals. *Obstet Gynecol* 1999;93(3):422-6.

8. Odent M. Is the participation of the father at birth dangerous? *Midwifery Today* 1999 (autumn); 51:23-4.

9. Terrence Real. *I don't want to talk about it. Overcoming the secret legacy of male depression.* Scribner NY 1997.

10. Odent M. Neonatal tetanus. *Lancet* 2008;371:385-386. doi:10.1016/S0140-6736(08)60198-1

Chapter 12

1. Kolås T, Saugstad OD, Daltveit AK, Nilsen ST, Øian P. Planned cesarean versus planned vaginal delivery at term: comparison of newborn infant outcomes. *Am J Obstet Gynecol* 2006 Dec;195(6):1538-43. Epub 2006 Jul 17.

2. Zanardo V, Padovani E, Pittini C, Doglioni N, Ferrante A, Trevisanuto D. The influence of timing of elective cesarean section on risk of neonatal pneumothorax. *J Pediatr* 2007 Mar;150(3):252-5.

3. Odent M. Vereinfachte Strategien im Zeitalter des vereinfachten Kaiserschnitts. In: *Der Kaiserschnitt: Indikationen. Hintergründe. Operatives Management der Misgav-Ladach-Methode* von Michael Stark von Urban & Fischer Verlag/Elsevier GmbH (Gebundene Ausgabe - 8. Dezember 2008).

Chapter 13

1. Csontos K, Rust M, Hollt V, et al. Elevated plasma beta-endorphin levels in pregnant women and their neonates. *Life Sci* 1979;25:835-44.

2. Akil H, Watson SJ, Barchas JD, Li CH. Beta-endorphin immunoreactivity in rat and human blood: Radioimmunoassay, comparative levels and physiological alterations. *Life Sci* 1979;24:1659-66.

3. Rivier C, Vale W, Ling N, Brown M, Guillemin R. Stimulation in vivo of the secretion of prolactin and growth hormone by beta-endorphin. *Endocrinology* 1977;100:238-41.

4. Heinrichs M, Meinlschmid G, Wippich W, et al. Selective

amnesic effects of oxytocin on human memory. *Physiol Behav* 2004;83(1):31–38.

5. Melzack R, Wall PD. Pain mechanisms: a new theory. *Science* 1965 Nov 19;150(699):971–979.

6. Odent M. La réflexothérapie lombaire. Efficacité dans le traitement de la colique néphrétique et en analgésie obstétricale. *La Nouvelle Presse Medicale* 1975;4(3):188.

7. Huntley AL, Coon JT, Ernst E Complementary and alternative therapies for labor pain: a systematic review. *Am J Obstet Gynecol* 2004 Jul;191(1):36-44.

8. Odent M. Birth under water. *Lancet* 1983;2:1476-7.

9. Eriksson M, Mattsson LA, Ladfors L. Early or late bath during the first stage of labour: a randomised study of 200 women. *Midwifery* 1997;13(3):146-48.

10. Norsk P, Epstein M. Effects of water immersion on arginine vasopressin release in humans. *J Appl Physiol* 1988;64(1): 1-10.

11. Gutkowska J, Antunes-Rodrigues J, McCann SM. Atrial natriuretic peptide in brain and pituitary gland. *Physiological Reviews* 1997;77(2):465-515. C-2

12. Mukaddam-Daher S, Jankowski M, et al. Regulation of cardiac oxytocin system and natriuretic peptide during rat gestation and postpartum. *J Endocrinol* 2002;175(1):211-6.

13. Gutkowska J, Jankowski M, et al. Oxytocin releases atrial natriuretic peptide by combining with oxytocin receptors in the heart. *Proc Nat Acad of Sci* USA 1997;94:11704-9.

14. Gilbert RE, Tookey PA. The perinatal mortality and morbidity among babies delivered in water. *BMJ* 1999; 319: 483-7.

15. Rosenear SK, Fox R, Marlow N. Stirrat GM. Birthing pools and the fetus. *Lancet* 1993; 342: 1048-9.

Chapter 14

1. Laborit H. 4-hydroxybutyrate. *Int J Neuropharmacol* 1964;32: 433-51.

2. Snead OC, Gibson M. Gamma-hydroxybutyric acid. NEJM 2005; 352:2721-32.

3. Odent M. Champagne and the fetus ejection reflex. *Midwifery Today* 2003 Spring;(65):9.

4. Santhakumar V, Wallner M, Otis TS. Ethanol acts directly on

extrasynaptic subtypes of GABAA receptors to increase tonic inhibition. *Alcohol* 2007; 41 (3): 211–21.

5. Liu SK, Fitzgerald PB, Daigle M, et al. The relationship between cortical inhibition, antipsychotic treatment, and the symptoms of schizophrenia. *Biol Psychiatry* 2009 Mar 15;65(6):503-9. Epub 2008 Oct 31.

6. Fattore L, Cossu G, Spano MS, et al. Cannabinoids and reward: interactions with the opioid system. *Crit Rev Neurobiol* 2004;16(1-2):147-58.

7. Kellogg CK, Yao J, Pleger GL. Sex-specific effects of in utero manipulation of GABA(A) receptors on pre- and postnatal expression of BDNF in rats. *Brain Res Dev Brain Res* 2000 Jun 30;121(2):157-67.

8. Kellogg CK, Kenjarski TP, Pleger GL, Frye CA. Region-, age-, and sex-specific effects of fetal diazepam exposure on the postnatal development of neurosteroids. *Brain Research* 2006 Jan 5;1067(1):115-25. Epub 2005 Dec 22.

9. Jacobson B, Nyberg K. Obstetric pain medication and eventual adult amphetamine addiction in offspring. *ACTA Obstet Gynecol Scand* 1988; 67:677-682.

10. Jacobson B, Nyberg K. Opiate addiction in adult offspring through possible imprinting after obstetric treatment. *BMJ* 1990;301:1067-70.

11. Nyberg K, Allebeck P, Eklund G, Jacobson, B. Socio-economic versus obstetric risk factors for drug addiction in offspring. *Br Addict* 1992; 87:1669-1676.

12. Nyberg K, Allebeck P, Eklund G, Jacobson, B. Obstetric medication versus residential area as perinatal risk factors for subsequent adult drug addiction in offspring. *Paediatr Perinatal Epidemiol* 1993;7: 23-32.

Chapter 15

1. Odent M. *The Farmer and the Obstetrician*. Free Association Books. London 2002.

2. Bentley-Lewis R. Gestational diabetes mellitus: an opportunity of a lifetime. *Lancet* 2009;373:1738-40.

3. Bellamy L, Casas J-P, Hingorani AD, Williams D. Type 2 diabetes mellitus after gestational diabetes: a systematic review and meta-analysis. *Lancet* 2009;373:1773-9.

4. Reece EA, Leguizamón G, Wiznitzer A. Gestational diabetes: the need for a common ground. *Lancet* 2009;373:1789-1797.
5. Odent M. Gestational diabetes and health promotion. *Lancet* 2009;374:684. doi:10.1016/S0140-6736(09)61555-5.
6. Wen SW, Liu S, Kramer MS, et al. Impact of prenatal glucose screening on the diagnosis of gestational diabetes and on pregnancy outcomes. *Am J Epidemiol* 2000;152(11):1009-14.
7. Thomas P, Golding J, Peters TJ. Delayed antenatal care: does it affect pregnancy outcome? *Soc Sci Med* 1991;32:715-23.
8. Douglas KA, Redman CW. Eclampsia in the United Kingdom. *BMJ* 1994;309:1395-400.
9. Vintzileos AM, Ananth CV, et al. The impact of prenatal care in the United States on preterm births in the presence or absence of antenatal high-risk conditions. *Am J Obstet Gynecol* 2002;187:1254-7.
10. Vintzileos AM, Ananth CV, et al. The impact of prenatal care on postneonatal deaths in the presence or absence of antenatal high-risk conditions. *Am J Obstet Gynecol* 2002; 187: 1258-62.
11. Binstock MA, Wolde-Tsadik G. Alternative prenatal care: impact of reduced visit frequency, focused visits and continuity of care. *J Reprod Med* 1995;40:507-12.
12. Sikorski J, Wilson J, et al. A randomised controlled trial comparing two schedules of antenatal visits: the antenatal project. *BMJ* 1996;312:546-53.
13. Villar J, Baaqueel H, et al. WHO antenatal care randomized trial for the evaluation of a new model of routine antenatal care. *Lancet* 2001;357:1551-64.
14. Wehbeh H, Matthews RP, et al. The effect of recent cocaine use on the progress of labor. *Am J Obstet Gynecol* 1995;172: 1014-8.
15. Ewigman BG, Crane JP, et al. Effect of prenatal ultrasound screening on perinatal outcome. *N Engl J Med* 1993;329:821-7.
16. Bucher HC, Schmidt JG. Does routine ultrasound scanning improve outcome in pregnancy? Meta-analysis of various outcome measures. *BMJ* 1993;307:13-17.
17. Larson T, Falck Larson J, et al. Detection of small-for-gestational-age fetuses by ultrasound screening in a high risk population: a randomized controlled study. *Br J Obstet Gynaecol* 1992;99:469-74.

18. Secher NJ, Kern Hansen P, et al. A randomized study of fetal abdominal diameter and fetal weight estimation for detection of light-for-gestation infants in low-risk pregnancy. *Br J Obstet Gynaecol* 1987;94:105-9.
19. Johnstone FD, Prescott RJ, et al. Clinical and ultrasound prediction of macrosomia in diabetic pregnancy. *Br J Obstet Gynaecol* 1996;103:747-54.
20. Steer P, Alam MA, Wadsworth J, Welch A. Relation between maternal haemoglobin concentration and birth weight in different ethnic groups. *BMJ* 1995;310:489-91.
21. Valberg LS. Effects of iron, tin, and copper on zinc absorption in humans. *Am J Clin Nutr* 1984;40:536-41.
22. Rayman MP, Barlis J, et al. Abnormal iron parameters in the pregnancy syndrome preeclampsia. *Am J Obstet Gynecol* 2002; 187(2):412-8.
23. Symonds EM. Aetiology of pre-eclampsia: a review. *J R Soc Med* 1980;73:871-75.
24. Naeye EM. Maternal blood pressure and fetal growth. *Am J Obstet Gynecol* 1981;141:780-87.
25. Kilpatrick S. Unlike pre-eclampsia, gestational hypertension is not associated with increased neonatal and maternal morbidity except abruptio. SPO abstracts. *Am J Obstet Gynecol* 1995; 419:376.
26. Curtis S, et al. Pregnancy effects of non-proteinuric gestational hypertension. SPO Abstracts. *Am J Obst Gynecol* 1995; 418: 376.

Chapter 17

1. Ewigman BG, Crane JP, et al. Effect of prenatal ultrasound screening on perinatal outcome. *N Engl J Med* 1993; 329: 821-7.
2. Bucher HC, Schmidt JG. Does routine ultrasound scanning improve outcome in pregnancy? Meta-analysis of various outcome measures. *BMJ* 1993;307:13-17.
3. Wen SW, Liu S, Kramer MS, et al. Impact of prenatal glucose screening on the diagnosis of gestational diabetes and on pregnancy outcomes. *Am J Epidemiol* 2000;152(11):1009-14.
4. International Association of Diabetes and Pregnancy Study Groups Recommendations on the Diagnosis and

Classification of Hyperglycemia in Pregnancy. *Diabetes Care.* 2010;33:676-683.

5.   Crowther CA, Hiller JE, Moss JR, McPhee AJ, Jeffries WS, Robinson JSL. Effect of treatment of gestational diabetes mellitus on pregnancy outcomes. *N Engl J Med* 2005;352:2477-86.

6.   Landon MB, Spong CY, Thom E, et al. A randomized trial of treatment for mild gestational diabetes. *N Engl J Med* 2009;361:1339-1348.

7.   Horvath K, Koch K, Jeitler K. Effects of treatment in women with gestational diabetes mellitus: systematic review and meta-analysis. *BMJ* 2010 Apr 1;340:c1395. doi: 10.1136/bmj. c1395.

INDEX